T0090255

HEALTH FOOD JUNKIES

Health Food JUNKIES

Overcoming the Obsession with Healthful Eating

Steven Bratman, M.D.,
with David Knight

Broadway Books
New York

BROADWAY

Broadway Books titles may be purchased for business or promotional use or for special sales. For information, please write to: Special Markets Department, Random House, Inc., 1540 Broadway, New York, NY 10036.

BROADWAY BOOKS and its logo, a letter B bisected on the diagonal, are trademarks of Broadway Books, a division of Random House, Inc.

Visit our website at www.broadwaybooks.com

Library of Congress Cataloging-in-Publication Data
Bratman, Steven.
Health food junkies: overcoming the obsession with healthful eating / Steven Bratman.
        p.   cm.
1. Eating disorders—Popular works.   2. Nutrition—Psychological aspects—Popular works.   3. Food habits—Psychological aspects—Popular works.   4. Junk food—Popular works.   5. Natural foods—Popular works.   I. Title.
RC552.E18   B73   2000
616.85'26—dc21
99-057249

Designed by Jennifer Ann Daddio

Interior photograph copyright 1999 Photodisk Inc.

ISBN 0-7679-0585-7

ISBN 978-0-767-90585-5

To Brother David,

whose generosity set me free

A c k n o w l e d g m e n t

Ellen Montague, M.S., M.A., L.P.C., whose critique and contributions make her in a real sense a coauthor.

Contents

SECTION 3

RECOVERY

HEALTH FOOD JUNKIES

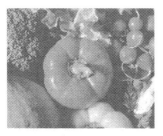

Introduction

Healing through nutrition is one of the pillars of alternative medicine. "Let your food be your medicine," the saying goes, and during my years of medical practice, patients have often begun their conversation with me by asking whether they can be cured through diet. I feel obliged to nod wisely. Although I am a conventionally trained M.D., I have been involved with alternative medicine since long before medical school, and a sacred reverence toward the healing power of diet is part of the job description of holistic physicians like myself. However, I am no longer the true believer in nutritional medicine I used to be. My own experience, as well as what I have seen happen to many of my patients, has affected me deeply. Too often I've seen the search for cure through diet become a disease worse than the original problem.

This book is about that disease, which I have named orthorexia nervosa. If you do not suffer from orthorexia yourself, the odds are high that a friend of yours does. Do you know anyone who seems to think constantly about choosing healthy food, who proselytizes some dietary theory supposed to cure all illnesses, who acts superior to other mortals who don't worry so much about eating? Have you run across raw-foodists and macrobiotic followers, or people who talk about food allergies, candida, or eating right for your blood type? I'd be very surprised if you haven't. Fascination with healing diets is increasingly common.

There have always been recommendations regarding the healthiest food to eat, but in recent decades the obsession over healthy eating seems to have escalated out of control. In more and more people it seems to be taking on the characteristics of an eating disorder like anorexia or bulimia. However, unlike these other eating disorders, orthorexia disguises itself as a virtue. Anorexics may know they are harming themselves, but orthorexics feel nothing but pride at taking care of their health in the best possible way.

I know how this feels, because I've been there myself. I've been at various times a raw-foodist, a total vegetarian, and a macrobiotic follower, and although I learned a lot from those experiences, it finally dawned on me that there is a dark side to dietary virtue. Similarly, as a holistic physician, I used to prescribe pure diets to my patients and only gradually came to understand that I wasn't necessarily doing them a favor. It's not that I don't support eating healthy food; it's only that when healthy eating becomes an obsession, it's no longer so healthy.

The good news is that orthorexia is not as difficult to cure as alcoholism, heroin addiction, or anorexia. The first section of this book tries to help the health food junkie admit that he or she really has a problem. The next section turns to some of the most common dietary theories that instigate orthorexia and shows that they are not the first and last word on health. Its purpose is to weaken the grip those theories can have on one's mind. Finally, the third part of this book gives specific advice on how to overcome orthorexia and learn again how to eat without obsession. It really is possible!

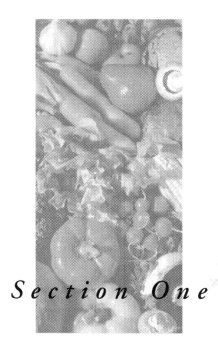

Section One

Understanding
ORTHOREXIA

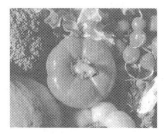

1.

What Is Orthorexia?

Twenty years ago I was a wholehearted, impassioned advocate of healing through food. My optimism was unbounded as I set forth to cure myself and everyone else. This was long before I became an alternative physician. In those days I was a cook and organic farmer at a large commune in upstate New York.

Like all communes in those days, ours attracted food idealists. I had to prepare several separate meals at once to satisfy the unyielding and contradictory dietary demands of those who inhabited our old Shaker village. The main entrée was invariably vegetarian. However, to placate a small but very insistent group, on an end table placed at some distance there could always be found a meat-based alternative. Actually, since at least 30 percent of our vegetarians refused to contemplate food cooked in pots and pans contaminated by fleshly vibrations, our burgers had to be prepared in a separate kitchen. The cooks also had to satisfy the vegans (non-dairy vegetarians), who looked on cheese as poison, as well as the non-garlic, non-onion, Hindu-influenced crowd, who believed that onion-family foods provoked sexual desire.

For the raw-foodists we laid out sliced raw vegetables in endless rows. Once, when a particularly enthusiastic visitor tried to convince me that slicing a vegetable would destroy its energy field, I felt so hassled that I ran at him wildly with a flat Chinese cleaver until he fled. Meanwhile, the macrobiotic followers condemned the raw vegetables for different theoretical reasons, and also set up a hue and cry over the serving of any "deadly nightshade" plants such as potatoes, tomatoes, and eggplants.

That wasn't all. Those who preferred choosing fruits and vegetables based on seasonal availability clashed violently with others who greedily demanded grapefruit in February.

Besides these widely varying opinions on which food to serve, there were as many theories on the method by which it should be prepared. Nearly all our food fanatics agreed that nothing should be cooked in an aluminum container, with the exception of our gourmet cooks, who explained that given our limited budget, only aluminum pots could spread the heat satisfactorily.

Everyone agreed that when steaming vegetables, only the minimum amount of water should be used, in order to save precious vitamins. The most severe enthusiasts would even hover around the kitchen toward the middle of food preparations and lay hands on the greenish liquids swirling at the bottom of the steamer. The matter of washing vegetables, however, remained swathed in controversy. Some commune members knew for a fact that the most nutritious portions of a vegetable lived in the skin. Others felt that a host of evil pollutants inhabited the same location, requiring exuberant scrubbing to detach. One visitor explained that the best policy was to dip all vegetables in bleach, giving out such a powerful line of reasoning for this course that we risked adopting the method on the spot. Luckily, we were out of bleach at that moment, and by the time we purchased some, the visitor—and the theory—had departed.

DIETARY EXTREMISM

The extremism of the above stories seems to be an inevitable complication of dietary theories. The crowning example in my memory occurred at a seminar held at the commune, led by a famous macrobiotic counselor I shall call Mr. Lux. An audience of at least thirty-five listened with rapt attention as Lux lectured on the evils of milk. "It slows the digestion," he explained, "clogs the metabolism, plugs the arteries, dampens the digestive fire, it causes mucus, respiratory diseases and cancer, and even sludges the soul so it can't see clearly."

At that time a member of the commune by the name of Matt lived in a small room upstairs from the seminar hall. He was a sometimes recovering alcoholic who rather frequently failed to abstain. Although he was only in his fifties, Matt's face showed the marks of a lifetime of alcohol abuse. He had been on the wagon for nearly six months when he tiptoed through the class.

Matt was a shy and private man. However, upon returning from the kitchen with a beverage, he discovered that there was no way he could reach his room without crossing through the crowded seminar. The leader noticed him immediately.

Pointing to the glass of milk in Matt's hand, Lux boomed out, "Don't you realize what that stuff is doing to your body, sir? Class, look at him! He is a testament to the health-destroying properties of milk. Study the puffy skin of his face. Note the bags under his eyes. Look at the stiffness of his walk. Milk, class—milk has done this to him!"

Bewildered, Matt looked at his glass, then up at the condemning faces, then back to the milk again. His lower lip quivered. "But," he whimpered, "but this is only milk, isn't it?"

In the Alcoholics Anonymous meetings with which Matt was familiar, cow's milk was practically mother's milk, synonymous with rectitude and purity. "I mean," he continued to the unforgiving students, "I mean, it isn't rum, is it?"

By focusing single-mindedly on diet and ignoring all other aspects of life, alternative practitioners like Mr. Lux come to practice a form of medicine that lacks a holistic perspective on life. This is ironic, of course, since holism is one of the strongest ideals of alternative medicine, at least as widely mentioned as healing through diet. It would be more holistic to take time to understand the whole person before making dietary recommendations and occasionally temper those recommendations with an acknowledgment of other elements in that person's life.

Unfortunately, patient and alternative practitioner too often work together to create an exaggerated focus on food. Rather than heal the person, this unbalanced emphasis can lead to a disease in its own right, the disease I call orthorexia. I know this disease well, because for many years I was one of the most extreme health-food fanatics you can imagine. In fact, I've come to think of it as a true eating disorder, not as life-threatening as bulimia and anorexia nervosa, but definitely in the same family.

ORTHOREXIA NERVOSA

To express this realization, I coined the term "orthorexia nervosa." It uses "ortho"—Greek meaning straight, correct, and true—to modify "anorexia nervosa." Orthorexia nervosa refers to a fixation on eating healthy food.

As we shall see later, there are often many hidden motivations behind orthorexia. But on the surface, at least, this eating disorder often begins innocently, as a desire to overcome chronic illness, lose weight, to improve general health, or to correct the many bad habits of the American diet. However, because it requires considerable willpower to adopt a diet that differs enormously from the food habits of one's culture, few can make the transition gracefully. Most of us resort to an iron self-discipline, often enhanced by a lofty feeling of superiority toward those who continue to eat a normal diet.

Over time, what to eat, how much, and the consequences of dietary indiscretion come to occupy a greater and greater proportion of our mental life. The effortful act of eating the right food may even begin to invoke a sense of spirituality. As orthorexia progresses, a day filled with wheat grass juice, tofu, and quinoa biscuits may come to feel as holy as one spent serving the destitute and homeless. On the other hand, when orthorexics fall off the path (which, according to the pertinent theory, may consist of anything from ingesting a single illegal raisin to devouring three quarts of Ben and Jerry's ice cream and a Big Mac), we experience it as a fall from grace. The only remedy is an act of penitence, which usually involves ever stricter diets or even fasting to cleanse away the influence of unhealthy foods.

This obsession seems silly to someone not so possessed. I've heard it called "kitchen spirituality," "cuisine dysfunction," and "food worship." But within the orthorexic there is a grim sense of self-righteousness that begins to consume all other sources of joy and meaning. An orthorexic will lose all pleasure at her child's birthday party because she has eaten a spoonful of ice cream along with the children; she will beat herself up for days over a slice of broccoli that was eaten cooked rather than raw.

Eventually orthorexia reaches a point at which the orthorexic devotes most of her life to planning, purchasing, preparing, and eating meals. If you had a window into her inner life, you'd see little else but self-condemnation for lapses, self-praise for success, strict self-control to resist temptation, and conceited superiority over anyone who indulges in impure dietary habits. The meaning of life has been displaced onto the bare act of eating.

It is precisely this displacement that defines orthorexia as an eating disorder. In this essential characteristic, orthorexia bears many similarities to the two named eating disorders: anorexia and bulimia. Whereas the bulimic and anorexic focus on the quantity of food, the orthorexic fixates on its quality. All three give to food a vastly excessive place in the scheme of life.

Proponents of nutritional medicine appear to remain blissfully unaware of the propensity for their theories to create an obsession. Indeed, popular books on natural medicine seem to actively promote orthorexia in their enthusiasm for sweeping dietary changes. No doubt, conventional medicine has made the opposite mistake, tending (until recently) to ignore the benefits of good diet. However, when healthy eating becomes a disease in its own right, it is arguably worse than the health problems that began the cycle of fixation.

MY OWN ESCAPE FROM ORTHOREXIA

I, too, passed through a phase of extreme dietary purity when I lived at the commune. In those days when I wasn't cooking, I managed the organic farm. This gave me constant access to fresh, high-quality produce. Eventually I became such a snob that I disdained to eat any vegetable that had been plucked from the ground more than fifteen minutes earlier. I was a total vegetarian, chewed each mouthful of food fifty times, always ate in a quiet place (which meant alone), and left my stomach partially empty at the end of each meal.

After a year or so of this self-imposed regime, I felt light, clear-headed, energetic, strong, and self-righteous. I regarded the wretched, debauched souls in the larger world around the commune, downing their chocolate chip cookies and fries, as mere animals reduced to satisfying gustatory lusts. But I wasn't complacent in my virtue. Feeling an obligation to enlighten my weaker brethren, I continuously lectured friends and family on the evils of refined, processed food and the dangers of pesticides and artificial fertilizers.

For two years I pursued wellness through healthy eating. Gradually, however, I began to sense that something was wrong. The need to obtain food free of animal products, fat, and artificial chemicals put nearly all social forms of eating out of reach. I began to sense that the poetry of my life had diminished. All I could think about was food.

But even when I became aware that my scrabbling in the dirt after raw vegetables and wild plants had become an obsession, I found it terribly difficult to free myself. I had been seduced by righteous eating. The center of my life's meaning had been transferred inexorably to food, and I could not reclaim it.

I was eventually saved from the doom of eternal health food

addiction through three fortuitous events. The first occurred when my guru, who was guiding me in the way of lacto-ovo-vegetarianism and was starting to tend toward fruitarianism, suddenly abandoned his quest. He explained that he had received a sudden revelation. "It came to me last night in a dream," he said. "Rather than eat my sprouts alone, it would be better for me to share a pizza with some friends." I looked at him dubiously, but I did not completely disregard his message.

The second event occurred when an elderly gentleman (whom I had been visiting as a volunteer home health aide) offered me a piece of Kraft Swiss cheese. Normally I wouldn't have considered accepting. I did not eat cheese, much less pasteurized, processed, and artificially flavored cheese. Worse still, I happened to be sick with a head cold that day. According to my belief system at that time, if I fasted, I would get over the cold in a day. However, if I allowed great lumps of indigestible dairy products to adhere to my innards, I would no doubt remain sick for a week—if I did not go on to develop pneumonia.

But Mr. Davis was earnest and persistent in his expression of gratitude, and he would have taken as a personal rebuke my refusal of the cheese. Shaking with trepidation, I chewed the dread processed product. To my great surprise, it seemed to have a healing effect. My cold symptoms disappeared within an hour. It was as if my acceptance of his gratitude healed me.

Nonetheless, even after this miracle I could not let go of my beliefs. I actually quit visiting Mr. Davis to avoid further defiling myself. That I would place food obsession over a human connection I truly valued filled me with shame, and now, as I look back, was a clear sign I was drowning.

The life preserver that finally drew me out was tossed by a

Benedictine monk named Brother David Stendl-Rast. I had met him at a seminar he gave on the subject of gratitude. Afterward, I volunteered to drive him home, for the purpose of getting to know him better. (This may be called "opportunistic volunteerism.") On the way to his monastery, although secretly sick of it, I bragged a bit about my oral self-discipline, hoping to impress the monk. I thought that he would respect me for never filling my stomach by more than half, and so on. David's actions were a marvelous example of teaching through action.

The drive was long. In the late afternoon we stopped for lunch at one of those out-of-place Chinese restaurants—the kind that flourish in small towns where it seems no one of remotely Asian ancestry has ever lived. As expected, all the waiters were Anglo-Saxon, but the food was unexpectedly good. The sauces were fragrant and tasty, the vegetables fresh, and the egg rolls crisp. We were both pleasantly surprised.

After I had eaten the small portion that sufficed to fill my stomach halfway, Brother David casually mentioned his belief that it was an offense against God to leave food uneaten on the table. This was particularly the case when such a great restaurant had so clearly been placed in our path as a special grace. David was a slim man and a monk, so I found it hardly credible that he followed this precept generally. But he continued to eat so much that I felt that good manners, if not actual spiritual guidance, required me to imitate his example. I filled my belly for the first time in a year.

Then he upped the ante. "I always think that ice cream goes well with Chinese food, don't you?" he asked blandly. Ignoring my incoherent reply, Brother David directed us to a Friendly's ice cream parlor and purchased me a triple-scoop cone.

David led me on a two-mile walk through the unexceptional

town as we ate our ice cream, edifying me with spiritual stories and in every way keeping my mind from dwelling on the Offense Against Health Food I had just committed. Later that evening Brother David ate an immense dinner in the monastery dining room, all the while urging me to have more of one dish or another. I understood the point. But what mattered more was the fact that this man, for whom I had the greatest respect, was giving me permission to break my health food vows. It proved a liberating stroke.

Yet it wasn't until more than a month later that I finally decided to make a decisive break. I was filled with feverish anticipation. Hordes of long-suppressed gluttonous desires, their legitimacy restored, clamored to receive their due. I set out from the commune toward the nearest junk food restaurant. On the twenty-minute drive into town, I planned and replanned my menu. Within ten minutes of arriving I had eaten three tacos, a medium pizza, and a large milkshake. I brought the ice cream sandwich and banana split home, for I was too stuffed to violate my former vows further. My stomach was stretched to my knees.

The next morning I felt guilty and defiled. Only the memory of Brother David kept me from embarking on a five-day fast (I fasted only two days). It took me many more years to attain the ability to follow a middle way in eating easily, without rigid calculation or wild swings. (See Section 3 for suggestions on how to accomplish this transition.)

Anyone who has ever suffered from anorexia or bulimia will recognize classic patterns in this story: the cyclic extremes, the obsession, the separation from others. These are all symptoms of an eating disorder. Having experienced them so vividly in myself twenty years ago, I cannot overlook their presence in others.

IS DIET A SIDE-EFFECT-FREE TREATMENT?

As an alternative physician, I often feel conflicted. I almost always recommend dietary improvements to my patients. How could I not? A low-fat, semivegetarian diet is potent preventive medicine for nearly all major illnesses, and more focused dietary interventions can often dramatically improve specific health problems. But I do not feel entirely innocent when I make dietary suggestions. I have come to regard dietary modification, like drug therapy, as a treatment with serious potential side effects.

Consider Andrea, a patient of mine who once suffered from chronic asthma. When she first came to see me, she depended on several medications to control her symptoms, but with my help she managed to free herself from all drugs. Yet I feel guiltier about my success with her than with any other patient I've seen while in practice.

The method we used involved identifying foods to which Andrea was sensitive and removing them from the diet. Milk was the first to go, then wheat, soy, and corn. After we'd eliminated those four foods, the asthma symptoms decreased so much that Andrea was able to cut out one medication. But she wasn't satisfied.

Diligent effort identified other allergens: eggs, avocado, tomatoes, barley, rye, chicken, beef, turkey, salmon, and tuna. These, too, Andrea eliminated, and she was soon able to drop another drug entirely. Next went broccoli, lettuce, apples, buckwheat, trout, and the rest of her medications.

Unfortunately, after about three months of feeling well, Andrea began to discover that there were now other foods to which she was sensitive. Oranges, peaches, celery, and rice didn't suit her, nor potatoes or amaranth biscuits. The only foods she could definitely tolerate were lamb and (strangely) white sugar. Since she couldn't actually live on only those foods, Andrea adopted a complex rotation diet, alternating grains on a meal-by-meal basis, with an occasional complete abstention to allow her to "clear." She did the same for vegetables, with somewhat more ease since there was a greater variety to choose from.

When Andrea came in for a follow-up visit a year later, her story disturbed me. Very pleased with the effects of diet but absolutely dependent on careful eating, Andrea carries a supply of her own particular foods wherever she goes. She doesn't go many places. Most of the time she stays at home thinking carefully about what to eat next, because when she slips up, the consequences endure for weeks. The asthma doesn't come back, but she develops headaches, nausea, and strange moods. She must continuously exert her will against cravings for foods as licentious as tomatoes and bread.

Andrea was happy with the treatment I'd given her, and she referred many of her friends to see me. Yet the sight of her name on my schedule continued to make me feel ill. The first rule of medicine is "Above all, do no harm." Have I helped Andrea by freeing her from drugs only to draw her into the bondage of diet? My conscience isn't clear.

If she had been cured of cancer or multiple sclerosis, I suppose that the development of an obsession wouldn't be too high a price for physical health. However, when we started treatment, all Andrea had was asthma. I have asthma, too. When she took her four medications, she had practically no asthma symptoms, and what's more, she had a life. Now all she has is a menu. Andrea might have been better off if she had never heard of dietary medicine.

I am generally lifted out of such melancholy reflections by some substantial success. The same day Andrea provoked that intense guilt, I saw Bob in follow-up, a man whose psoriatic arthritis (a rather unusual and often quite painful form of arthritis) was thrown into full remission by two simple interventions: removing wheat from his diet and adding foods high in trace minerals. Before he met me, he took dangerously high doses of prednisone. After we started, he needed no medications at all. Seeing him encouraged me not to give up entirely on making dietary recommendations.

But my enthusiasm remains tempered. Like all other medical interventions—like all other solutions to difficult problems—dietary medicine dwells in a gray zone of unclarity and imperfection. It's neither a simple, ideal treatment, as some of its proponents believe, nor the complete waste of time conventional medicine has too long presumed it to be. Diet is an ambiguous and powerful tool, too unclear and emotionally charged for comfort, too powerful to be ignored.

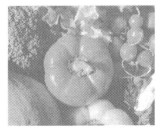

2.

A Disease Disguised as a Virtue

In Western Europe and America we abuse our abundance of food and eat badly. As a group, we consume too much meat and fat and eat too few whole grains and fresh fruits and vegetables. Empty calories make up such a high percentage of our diets that, while growing overweight, we nonetheless don't get all the vitamins and minerals we need. It certainly makes sense to change our dietary habits, exercise self-discipline, and learn to eat in ways that that will keep us healthier longer. Studies organized by researchers such as Dean Ornish have shown just how profoundly we can improve our health by choosing more carefully what to put on our plate.

It is certainly not the point of this book to dispute the value of healthy diet. Proper food choices can clearly reduce the risk of cancer and heart disease, and may be able to prevent other major illnesses of middle and later life. This is a well-known and incontestable fact. What I do want to point out, however, is that there is a dark side to this reality, an unintended consequence of the emphasis on eating properly. There is more to life than reducing cancer risk. Too often this holistic perspective is forgotten by those who emphasize that food is the best medicine.

In the process of adding extra years to our lives, we can make our lives meaningless. Does it make sense to use food to prolong life while devoting that life primarily to food? Such a circle of meaninglessness is surprisingly common. Focus becomes obsession, self-discipline becomes self-punishment, and effort itself can turn into an addiction. The quest for healthy food can become a disease in its own right, as bad in a way as the diseases it is meant to forestall or cure. To take a cue from the popular bumper sticker, LIFE IS TOO SHORT TO DRINK BAD WINE, life is too short to spend it all thinking about how to live longer.

This is the contrarian premise of this book: Obsession with healthy diet is an illness, an eating disorder. Unlike anorexia, it seldom kills anyone (although I have seen it happen), but it is a dead end, a trap, a backwater. Amid all the hyperbole about eating healthy food, all the compelling arguments for one dietary theory or another, this reality has been ignored by those who should know better. The same people who profess to endorse holistic health have spent decades encouraging people to neglect their other needs in favor of dietary obsession.

You can throw away your life by trying to save it. It happens all the time, and ironically, you can pat yourself on the back the whole way down the path to the cliff's edge and over it. I did it for years. I was full of self-congratulation, full of superiority for those wretches out there eating the wrong food, all the while making my own life empty and meaningless.

For almost twenty-five years I have been involved with what is variously called alternative medicine, natural medicine, or holistic medicine. I became a food fanatic shortly after discovering the concept of natural foods, and during my years of professional practice I met thousands of individuals whose defining interest in life was eating according to one or another theory. Over time the craziness of this lifestyle began to dawn on me, while simultaneously I began to notice just how arbitrary, puritanical, and contradictory the various food theories really were. I began to find myself more often trying to talk my patients out of strict diets than into them.

But I found that people who had been trapped by intense food faiths were very difficult to set free. Dietary theories carry the gravity of religion. If I directly confronted the sacred beliefs of Health Food Theory A or B, I would be perceived as an infidel, an evildoer, an agent of the medical/agricultural/dairy industry. I found that it required a bit of a devious approach to make any headway. I had to begin with full sympathy and apparent support for the dietary theory in question. Only later could I begin to chip away at the foundation of the theory to loosen its hold. The need for subtlety was even true for those who were ready to break free, who wanted to relax a bit and stop obsessing over what they ate. Any direct approach activated the articles of faith and acted to strengthen the obsession rather than weaken it.

I gradually discovered that a light, humorous tone worked best, one that gently mocked the tenets of food religion in order to loosen its imperious grip. I started to look for ways to make the apparent virtue of cuisine righteousness appear more realistically as a vice, or a psychological disorder. My improvisations in this direction began to meet with some success. By the early 1990s I would guess that I worked with orthorexic tendencies in about half the people in my medical practice.

In 1994 I began to look actively for a medical-sounding word to describe health food obsession. I started out with the misapprehension that most medical terms were phrased in Latin, and so I contacted Latin scholars. One came up with the term *"cupiditas cibi salubrum,"* meaning "craving for healthy food." It sounded nice but didn't resemble any other diagnostic term I'd ever heard. I then discovered that Greek was the actual language of medical diagnostics and was soon told that a good expression might be "ortho-orexia nervosa." "Ortho" means "right" or "correct," as in "orthogonal" (right angle); "orexia" relates to eating or appetite, as in "anorexia" ("no appetite"). "Nervosa" simply means "obsession" or "fixation." With the permission of my scholars, I removed the repeated O and made it "orthorexia nervosa."

To be perfectly honest, I intended the term somewhat tongue in cheek, as a kind of sassy way to surprise clients who were proud of their obsession and make them think twice about it. I assumed that the condition was fairly rare and that the only reason I saw it so often was that I practiced alternative medicine. Food obsession seemed to be a sixties and seventies problem, lingering only in those for whom the experience of those decades continued to be a major part of their lives, a problem endemic to the same demographic that would buy the new VW bugs. But I was not quite right.

When I used the term "orthorexia nervosa" in an article for *Yoga Journal*, later reprinted in *The Utne Reader*, the response was unexpectedly intense. A prominent yoga teacher called to say, "You woke me up with a jolt. I thought I was the best eater in the county; after I read your article, I realized that even to think that way is a form of insanity."

A junior high school teacher from Illinois wrote, "Underneath my pride, I think I knew there was something pretty nuts about thinking about food all day. Your article pinned me like a butterfly.

It made me look at myself, and what I see isn't pretty. I've been using healthy food to hide from everything else."

Perhaps the most plaintive note read, "If I don't pay such close attention to food, what am I going to think about all day long?" This anonymous writer said he was an air-traffic controller. I certainly hoped he was able to spare some of his attention for airplanes! I hadn't realized how widely orthorexia is distributed throughout modern society. My correspondents ranged in age from fourteen to seventy-nine and included a state congressman, a policewoman, a veterinarian, and three big-rig truck drivers. Letters came from Europe and Japan as well as the United States.

Ironically, about one-third of these respondents missed my point. They requested information on exactly what extreme diet they should choose to cure their health problems. "I would like to use the orthorexia you describe to cure my knee pain," one caller said. "I've already cut out all deadly-nightshade vegetables, grains, sugar, caffeine, meat, and nuts. Do you think I should go on a water fast one week each month?"

However, some food fanatics did understand. The manager of an Internet site for raw foods called to admit that I had touched a chord. "We in the raw foods movement need to remember that there is more to life than food," he said. "My readers need to see this perspective." He posted my article on his Web site, provoking a storm of excitement that included both appreciation and violent attacks. For daring to confront the health food gods, I was accused by some readers of being in league with agribusiness and the ten evil men who rule the world. "You just want to sell beef and dairy," one wrote. But others seemed to be touched by what they read. "I think Bratman may be on to something," said one post. "Maybe I do take food too seriously."

Some people rather amusingly used my article to bash their enemies. "I agree with you completely," said one note. "Those people who won't even eat raw grains are over the top. Me, I like to loosen up now and then and eat some raw millet and amaranth." Another wrote, "Your devastating critique of the 'health food' movement amused me greatly. People who make up arbitrary dietary restrictions instead of following the true laws of eating are really crazy."

Later, a food reporter for *Cosmopolitan* magazine wrote a story on the subject. The response to her article was, in her words, "the biggest reaction I have had to any food column." Obsessive food-allergy avoidance seemed to be the most common dietary excess of *Cosmo* readers who found my number and called, although non-dairy vegetarianism, fruitarianism, and a kind of anorexia/orthorexia were also surprisingly common. A few months later, *Spin* magazine ran an article on the raw foods revival, and although they didn't use the term "orthorexia," it was clear from the article that the food ideals I had thought peculiar to the sixties were making a whole new generation of converts. The misguided impulse to find happiness in health food has surprising staying power.

IS HEALTHY EATING
ALWAYS ORTHOREXIA?

Despite everything I say in this book, I do not mean to imply that you should simply eat junk, that to make healthy dietary choices is a disease. It's the quality of obsession that defines orthorexia, not the desire to eat healthy food; it's the absence of moderation, the loss of perspective and balance, the transfer of too much of life's meaning onto food. When diet becomes an escape from life, it begins to resemble an eating disorder more than a sensible choice.

It's easy to find a comparison in anorexia nervosa. The desire to avoid excessive weight is perfectly reasonable. If a person chooses to count calories in order to fight a tendency toward obesity and exercises regularly to maintain muscle tone, that's simply a healthy decision. It's only when this impulse takes on a life of its own that we would define it as a problem; when a person exercises and diets down to eighty or ninety pounds she has lost perspective and balance, and it is fair to call her behavior an eating disorder.

The same is the case with orthorexia. When a sense of compulsion begins to override free choice, when you begin to judge everyone else on the basis of diet rather than on character or personality, when you spend many of your waking hours thinking about food, you are not simply making dietary choices. You are not a virtuous eater. You have an eating disorder.

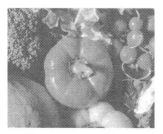

3.

The Dangers
of Orthorexia

Anorexia, we know, is a disease that kills by starvation. Some treatment programs for anorexia require participants to eat at least one full meal under supervision, and sometimes only tube feeding can sustain life. But how can addiction to health food harm you? It's *healthy* food, after all. It should be good for you.

But anything becomes unhealthy when pursued without a sense of balance. The obsessive nature of orthorexia frequently leads to a loss of all sense of proportion and an inexorable progression toward greater extremes of diet. As we will see in later chapters, raw-foodism becomes fruitarianism (eating only fruit) and finally breatharianism (trying to live on air alone—I am not kidding). The macrobiotic diet starts with brown rice, beans, and vegetables and progresses to brown rice alone. Food-allergy diets can lead to eating nothing but turkey, sweet potatoes, and white rice. In advanced cases orthorexia can lead to significant malnutrition, causing susceptibility to severe infections and the potential for death. Although such cases are not common, I have seen several, and they represent orthorexia at its worst.

Even when orthorexia does not involve a diet so extreme as to be physically dangerous, it can cause a subtler problem, a kind of psychological malnutrition as emotionally disabling as other psychological diseases. Even if a person doesn't die from obsessive-compulsive disease, depression, or chronic anxiety, these are clearly psychological illnesses that need treatment. The same is true of orthorexia. This disease causes a drastic shrinking of life's options and is all the more insidious in that the orthorexic typically feels proud of his or her lifestyle.

DEATH BY ORTHOREXIA

In its worst form orthorexia takes on a similarity to anorexia, in that it leads to a kind of deliberate starvation. Orthorexia this intense is hard to miss.

When Martha called me, there were obvious notes of terror in her voice.

"I wonder if my friend could have that disease you're talking about," she said. "Sometimes I think I should call the police. If she dies, and I don't do anything about it . . . Don't you have an obligation sometimes?"

I asked her what food habits of her friend worried her.

"She doesn't eat anything."

"You mean she's a breatharian?"

"What's that?"

"Someone who tries to live only on air."

"Thank God, Janice isn't that bad. Breatharian? That's got to be a joke."

"No, it isn't. But tell me about Janice."

"Every week it's something else she can't eat. Now it's gluten, so wheat is out. Last month it was dairy, and it's still dairy."

"So far your story doesn't scare me," I said. "People can be allergic to gluten, wheat, and dairy products. Many people eliminate those foods from their diet and feel better for it."

At this point in the conversation, I wasn't sure whether it was Martha or her friend who had a problem. It's easy to criticize the way another person eats; it's even easy to get passionate about it. At least a dozen times I've attempted to protect people whose relatives or friends wanted to "rescue" them from a balanced, healthy vegetarian diet. I always wonder about the motives of someone who wants to change another person's diet (even when I'm the one who is doing it). It's similar to fixing another person's marriage. Unless a diet (or a marriage) goes over a certain line, an outsider really doesn't have the right to intervene.

But Martha settled my doubts in a hurry. "All she eats right now, I think, is Jerusalem artichoke pasta, canola oil, and watermelon."

That didn't sound good. "Does she have a doctor recommending these strict dietary changes?"

"That's the problem—she does have a doctor, and the *doctor* is scared. He got the ball rolling last spring when he gave her an allergy test. But now he's pronounced her well enough to go back to eating a normal diet. The scary thing is that she won't believe him. She said he'd 'gone straight' on her, and she stopped going to his office."

I took note that the direct approach was not likely to work with Janice.

"Does she eat any protein?" I asked. "Nuts, beans, tofu—anything like that?"

"Beans give her gas, tofu is too processed, and as for nuts . . .

well, she says they *make* you nuts, and that's how they got the name. Her muscles have melted down to nothing. I think she's starving herself."

This story brought back memories of when I had been so extreme about my own diet that I began to look like a concentration camp victim. Martha must have caught something of my thoughts, because she became more agitated. "It's just as if she had anorexia," she said. "If I don't get her into treatment, I'm afraid she's going to die. She's a wonderful person, too. She's just gotten crazy on account of her diet."

Because I was an alternative doctor, Janice was happy to come see me, no doubt imagining that I would advise her on more foods not to eat. When I saw her, I was appalled. She weighed about ninety-five pounds, and since she was five and a half feet tall, this wasn't good. Her cheeks sank in so far I found myself wondering whether they met in the middle, and her arms seemed like bones with a mere halo of skin.

For me, the meeting was tense. It seemed to me a real possibility that legally I might be obliged to hospitalize her against her will, as one might do with someone suicidal. But if I did, she would certainly never trust me again, or Martha. I considered other possibilities while outwardly maintaining a neutral demeanor. After about twenty minutes I finally conceived a rather desperate plan. It involved feigning an enthusiasm I didn't feel, but I couldn't think of any other solution to her problem.

I started talking about macrobiotics in such a way as to make it sound like the most fascinating imaginable approach to healing.

"Food allergies don't get to the root of the problem," I said, using a famous line from alternative medicine. "It's just a Band-Aid solution. Yes, I understand that you are allergic to wheat. But *why* are you allergic to wheat? Simply avoiding the food doesn't solve anything, now, does it?" I went on to explain how macrobiotics could get to the root of her problem, really heal her from within.

If I had directly criticized her diet, I would have immediately lost all rapport with Janice. But by my using this indirect approach, Janice could hear me. Within a week she had abandoned her previous food beliefs to take up macrobiotics. It's not that I am a follower of macrobiotics. As I describe in Chapter 8, that dietary theory has its own set of problems. However, macrobiotics is a definite step up from the way Janice was eating; it would certainly keep her alive.

Janice's orthorexia was the most dangerous kind, because it contained so many elements of anorexia. She was focused on *removing* foods from her diet; the less she ate, the better she felt about herself. This is very common among those who follow food allergy theories. It is equally common in raw-foodism, which shares a great many psychological similarities to anorexia. (See Chapter 7 for more information.) Macrobiotics, on the other hand, encourages obsession with diet, but except for short periods of time it involves eating enough food and in sufficient variety to maintain health.

I tried the same tactics with Diana, another food allergy believer who was starving herself to death, but this time I failed. The idea of macrobiotics intrigued her, but she couldn't stand the experience of having something as heavy as brown rice in her stomach. Like so many orthorexics (and anorexics, for that matter), she was addicted to the feeling of physical lightness. Brown rice seemed to weigh her down too much; it gave her unmistakable evidence of existing in a body, and she was one of those who had opted for feeling like some kind of angel of light. Diana went back to her usual diet of white rice and lamb; became vitamin- and mineral-malnourished; successfully eluded her friends, doctors, and civil authorities who planned to hospitalize her; and eventually died of the flu. Her body was just too malnourished to defend itself against the virus.

Another patient of mine died the same year. Brenda was a rawfoods fanatic who ate only fruits and vegetables. Although her diet provided plenty of vitamins and minerals, there was precious little protein in it, and she kept fainting. She successfully talked me into not hospitalizing her by promising to eat some nuts and legumes, but within days of this promise she crashed her car into the front of a store and died. She is believed to have fainted while driving.

The third death was a woman who also ate only raw vegetables. Her belly swelled up like that of a starving Biafran child (proteincalorie malnutrition causes a swollen belly), and she died in a motel room, hiding out from the friends who wanted to hospitalize her.

I've heard at least six other stories of death by orthorexia, one of them going back to that first bloom of vegetarianism, the 1920s. Keep in mind, however, that these cases are fairly rare. Most probably represent an overlap of orthorexia and anorexia. Usually orthorexia won't kill you; its harm lies in what it does to the mind and spirit, the way it creates a distorted and unhealthy view of life.

PRIORITIES UPSIDE DOWN

The most usual harm caused by orthorexia is the cost of lost opportunities. Life is too short to spend our waking hours thinking about nothing but food. The distorted priorities of orthorexia stem from an obsession that makes food seem much more important than it really is; while obsessed with food, we miss numerous chances for greater life.

Obsessiveness is part of the very nature of orthorexia. In fact, if you eat a healthy diet but don't obsess over it, if you follow dietary guidelines effortlessly and focus most of your energy on living life, you almost certainly don't have orthorexia. You just eat well. It's the forcefulness, the overdetermined nature of orthorexia, that constitutes an illness.

We have all experienced some degree of obsession. When we really want something, we can't think about anything else, even if we try. It's as if we're in love. Think of the words to every love song ever written. "You are my everything." "I can't live if living is without you." "You are the sun and the moon to me."

Of course we can "live" without the object of our affection, and nobody really is our "everything." Yet when we are in love, these words ring as true as true can be. It's the same with orthorexia. We concentrate entirely on how healthy our food is, and diet becomes the most important thing in the world. We are in love with food, in a state of high romance with a vegetable. There are probably better places to put that energy.

Love for another human being is important. It's one of the major experiences of life. The passion to be near your loved one, to do things together, to talk to and about each other has been celebrated in movies, books, and poems throughout recorded history.

Not so the passion to eat healthy food. This is a dead-end love affair. When orthorexia begins to push out all other interests in your life, it is not a lovely romance: it is a mistake, like going to the theater and spending the whole evening hooked on a video game in the bathroom.

Orthorexia won't kill you; in most cases it won't even cause permanent physical damage. But it is just as disabling, in its own way, as a serious emotional illness. Our friends may say, "Look at what you're doing to yourself. Wake up! Quit it!" Unfortunately, this self-imposed deprivation usually looks perfectly sensible from within.

Consider Claire, a young woman who came to David Knight for psychotherapy a couple of years ago. She badly wanted to be in a relationship, but since her divorce she hadn't been able to find the right person. She habitually chose men who weren't very interested in her, and she would work frantically to make them love her.

As therapy progressed, Claire came to realize that she was seeking relationships in the wrong way. She was looking for "trophies," men who she thought would make her look good rather than men she really loved. She worked diligently in therapy to overcome this tendency, and she seemed to be making good progress.

Claire was also a bit of a health fanatic. She spent at least fifteen minutes of each therapy session talking about how well she'd eaten that week. David didn't see any problem with this. Today, he says, he can spot orthorexia from ten miles off. Back then he just saw her dietary obsession as healthy self-care.

Nine months after therapy began, Claire met a man who didn't fit the mold of her previous relationships. Brian was not incredibly good-looking, rich, or famous. But she really liked him. He was sensitive, talked about his feelings, and didn't keep her at a distance the way other men had. For a change she was with someone who seemed to care as much about her as she did for him. Everything seemed to be going well, until the day she came into the office and exclaimed, "It's over."

As David tells it, "She must have seen the surprise on my face, because she explained, 'He smelled bad.' "

Being the ever-insightful therapist who is never surprised by anything, David sputtered, "What? . . . Huh?"

"He smelled bad because he drank coffee," she went on. "First thing every day he gets up and pours that poison down his throat. I thought I could get him to change, but he won't. I can't stand the smell of it on his breath anymore, and even worse, I don't get how he can treat his body so badly. He even puts sugar in his coffee. This man is not for me."

"Uh . . . what?" David responded with the best psychotherapeutic technique he could muster at the moment.

"Look," Claire told him, "he was nice and everything, but how could I possibly think about having a future with someone who is so unhealthy? I would have to supervise him all the time to make sure that he wasn't poisoning himself. And as soon as I took my eyes off him, he would go out and get a cup. It's like he's unconscious."

Claire really wanted a partner, but her food obsessions were more powerful. Keeping certain foods out of her life was more important than love. She gave up on a potentially wonderful relationship, not because the guy was insensitive or cold or an alcoholic. He just didn't fit into her particular food obsession.

From the outside this story might sound crazy. But Claire isn't crazy. She's just obsessed with food.

I recall a time when it was an absolute criterion for my choice of possible mates that she be a vegetarian. If I went out on a date and found that a woman used mayonnaise or ate white bread or drank sodas, we might still be friends (in a distant sort of way), but true intimacy was clearly out of the question.

In retrospect, I see that this was an insane yardstick. How can dietary preference rank as an important consideration, as compared to character, kindness, interests, emotional maturity, sense of values? A difference in diet might present some challenges in developing a weekly menu, but when we make decisions on whom to marry and whom to befriend based on it, something has gone wrong.

I sometimes use an "end of my life" test to evaluate my priorities. It works like this: Imagine yourself lying on your deathbed and remembering the years that have passed. Then visualize whatever decision you are considering, and look at it from the perspective of the end of your life.

I did this once sometime after rejecting a woman based on her diet. I tried to imagine myself saying, "I'm so glad I never dated X. Yes, she was loving, deep, sensitive, mature, a real human being. But she ate meat. My life is much richer for having rejected her on that basis."

Not likely.

ORTHOREXIA AND OBSESSIVE-COMPULSIVE DISORDER

Beyond a general obsession with food and the resulting distortion of priorities, orthorexia frequently goes further and shares dramatic similarities with obsessive-compulsive disorder (OCD). This psychological condition was made famous by Jack Nicholson in the movie *As Good as It Gets*. Nicholson displays many of the classic behavior patterns of those with this emotional illness. His character needs to open a new bar of soap each day, washes his hands obsessively, compulsively checks and rechecks his house before going anywhere to see if he's forgotten anything, and obsesses over where he sits in a restaurant.

All but the most carefree among us suffer from obsessive habits to some extent, but in OCD this impulse takes on a life of its own and becomes a real handicap. Orthorexia sometimes seems to be a form of this disorder, with numerous overlapping and similar features.

For example, Nicholson feels the need to bring his own silverware to restaurants. This is very much like the orthorexic's need to bring his own food everywhere he goes. Other habits of orthorexics are even more blatantly obsessive: the need experienced by followers of various dietary theories to carefully weigh and measure all the foods and liquids they consume, the focus on planning meals, the guilt over any deviation from the dietary plan, and even the very preoccupation with food itself all look strikingly like obsessive-compulsive disease.

When I look back at the years of my own fixation on healthy eating, I see glaring patterns of obsessiveness, some of which are rather embarrassing to recall. For example, I used to get "stuck" in the natural food store, unable to decide exactly what to purchase for lunch. I would wake up in the morning thinking about dinner and at night plan what I was going to eat (or not eat) for the next several days. These are all clearly obsessive patterns. But the evening with the avocado was the most extreme, and even in the midst of it I knew that something was out of control.

The avocado incident took place after dinner, in a house that I shared with friends in Santa Cruz. Although they were only friends, at that particular moment we all felt like family. We were having one of those wonderful warm conversations that doesn't come often enough in life: as engaging as an argument and as amicable as Christmas dinner on a TV show from the fifties. I wanted it to go on forever. Unfortunately, an avocado was calling to me from the fruit bowl. I knew that if I answered the call, our party would start to break up, but I couldn't put it out of my mind.

I had purchased that avocado three days previously, and I'd carefully examined and turned it every day since. The morning of our dinner party, I had determined that it needed another half day, and although I'd forgotten about it for a while, I suddenly recalled that it was ripe and needed attention.

I imagined the bright green color of its meat, shading lighter toward the center. As yet it would have no dark streaks or stringy fibers; as yet it radiated life energy. But tomorrow it would begin the downward slide into decay that meant eating it would rob my body of energy rather than feeding it.

Someone was talking to me. I tore my mind away from the avocado and answered her. Everyone laughed at what I said, freeing me to think once more about the avocado.

If I got it into the refrigerator immediately and ate it tomorrow at lunch, its radiant glow would penetrate my cells, healing me, helping me to fight off the flu that was going around. I reached out toward it but pulled back my hand when someone asked me a question. The avocado receded. I sipped my spring water and made another funny comment, meanwhile grabbing the avocado and pulling it into my lap. I squeezed it slightly. It was perfect. Could I just get up, put it in the refrigerator, and come back without disturbing the evening?

I knew it wouldn't work. If I got up, everyone would get up.

I tried to forget the avocado, to put it in perspective. I'd been feeling lonely for months. Tonight it felt as if I had a family; I felt as if I belonged. It was crazy to think about a stupid avocado at a time like this.

But I couldn't stop fiddling with it. Even now its bright green cells were turning brown, one by one, its life force dwindling as decay set in. I squeezed it again, realizing that by doing so I was increasing its need for refrigeration. All along the dents I might make, its cells would start to change, their lining damaged by the displacement.

I stood up smoothly and walked to the kitchen. I opened the

refrigerator and quickly slid the avocado onto the first shelf. Could I get back before . . . ?

People were standing up. In minutes the party was over. I had blown it. I felt lonely.

I took the avocado from the refrigerator, hesitated, and then cut into it. It was perfect. I could almost pretend that I wasn't lonely as I ate it.

While this was far from the first time I'd been obsessed with food, it was one of the clearest incidents in which I recognized that the obsession was troubling. Too often I had been proud and happy to be obsessed! Now I realized that it was making me miserable. The transition from unconscious acceptance of obsessiveness to awareness of a desire to break free from it is one of the hallmarks of change; it is the first step to freedom.

Looking at it honestly, we can see that the obsessiveness of orthorexia defeats its original justification anyway. By distorting our priorities and upsetting the balance of our lives, orthorexia actually makes us sicker rather than healthier. To be really healthy we have to relax, live a little, flow with the movements of life, not grasp frantically after a perfect diet.

ORTHOREXIA AND SOCIAL ISOLATION

One of the primary features of orthorexia is the feeling that we are better than others because of our fantastic diet. Since the rest of the world does not adhere to the God-given laws of healthy eating (as we uniquely understand them), we can't eat with the rest of the world. Besides, a great deal of our identity is tied up in diet. We may perceive political implications to what we eat; we also may enjoy the role of being an outsider and use food to shore up the wall between us and the outside world.

The net effect is social isolation. The ancient satisfaction of breaking bread with a friend is denied us; we must either bring our own bread (a concoction of potato flour, amaranth, and spelt that only an orthorexic could love) or eat alone. This isolation is a real emotional harm caused by orthorexia. (Or we may use orthorexia as an excuse to isolate ourselves. See Chapter 16, "Identifying Hidden Agendas.") As my health food guru realized in Chapter 1, "Rather than eat my sprouts alone, it would be better for me to share a pizza with some friends." A good half or more of the joy of life comes from relationships; when orthorexia interferes with those relationships, it causes a real impoverishment of our lives.

Not only does it damage us emotionally, social isolation also causes physical harm. Good scientific evidence tells us that the strength of our social connections is a significant factor in our ability to survive and avoid illnesses. By fostering separation from others, orthorexia defeats its own purpose, and worsens rather than improves our health.

ORTHOREXIA AND CHILDREN

If you read books on natural health, you will find yourself encouraged to believe that fostering healthy dietary habits in your children is practically the most virtuous step you can take in life. No doubt, it is wise to teach our children to eat properly. But this laudatory desire can easily create one of the most troubling scenarios of orthorexia: transmission of the disease to a child by a parent who has become "infected" with orthorexia. It's bad enough when a parent is obsessed, but when I see a child whose little life is wrapped obsessively around food, I want to burn all the books on natural medicine for children.

The story of Shirley and her six-year-old daughter, Jane, is one of the most painful of my career. I've seen many similar cases, but this was the most personally troubling. Shirley came to me for treatment of her migraine headaches. She brought Jane along to the appointment, too. Jane leaned on her mother's knee and joined eagerly in the conversation, which went somewhat as follows:

> SHIRLEY: My headaches have been better since I discovered food allergies, but I still get them every couple of months.
> MYSELF: How often did you used to get them?
> SHIRLEY: Nearly every day. Jane had migraines, too, until I took her off dairy, wheat, fruit, oatmeal, vegetable oils, sugar, peanut butter, corn, and eggs.

Quite a list for a six-year-old, I thought. And why did she switch subjects to her daughter?

> MYSELF: Were Jane's headaches as bad as yours?
> JANE: They were worser than my mom's.
> SHIRLEY *(laughing):* Well, not as bad as mine, sweetheart. *(Now she turned to me.)* I don't think she ever actually had headaches, not real ones, you know. But I could tell she was about to have a bad headache. Her mood would change, just like mine does. I get so irritable when I'm about to have a headache. I didn't want her to go through the same thing as me, so I started treating her even before she had any headaches. Prevention, you know.

MYSELF: Well, prevention is a great concept. *(I wanted to tell her to quit projecting her own health problems on her daughter.)* How often does she get irritable?

JANE: Whenever I eat bad foods, I get really, really grumpy.

SHIRLEY: It used to be that she'd get angry all the time. Over nothing.

MYSELF: Give me an example.

SHIRLEY: Well, supposing we went shopping for a couple of hours at the mall. If I didn't get her something, she'd start whining, "It's not fair, you're getting to buy things. I should get to buy them, too."

MYSELF: Sounds reasonable to me.

SHIRLEY: Oh, but it wasn't Jane. Jane is a perfect little kid. She never whines about anything. Not unless it's her food allergies getting to her. Isn't that right, Jane?

JANE: Yesterday I yelled at my friend Ashley when she wouldn't let me on the seesaw. It was because I had chocolate.

SHIRLEY: That stupid teacher gave her chocolate earlier in the week. I knew something would happen, and sure enough, two days later she yells at her friend. Her best friend! Can you imagine that? You're not ever supposed to yell at your friends.

JANE *(shaking her head):* Never yell at your friends.

SHIRLEY: It's just the chocolate that made her do it. We're both the same that way. The other day I yelled at my sister—it was because I had a diet soda.

My heart was aching. What a way to raise a child! To believe that every natural emotion is the consequence of a dietary indiscretion, that to get angry is a physical imbalance, that to feel annoyed at one's friends or relatives is an aberration that must be corrected by more diligent application of a dietary theory—it's a recipe for building a person totally ignorant of his or her real nature as a human being.

What could I do? I couldn't say to Jane, "Your mother has an obsession, and she's indoctrinating you with it." I would have to address the mother, and I knew it would be an extremely delicate subject.

I didn't say anything about it for the first several visits. Instead we concentrated on acupuncture, osteopathic manipulation, and other therapeutic methods. With each successive visit it seemed that we were building more trust. Finally I judged that the time was right to put out a feeler.

"Do you think it's ever possible to be too focused on diet?" I asked Shirley.

"No," she said.

That was a stopper, but I tried again.

"I mean, do you suppose that sometimes diet isn't the cause of a health problem?"

"Oh," she said, standing up. "You think I'm a health fanatic, too. I should have known." Casting me a vicious look and waving aside any attempt to explain, she left, taking her daughter with her.

She then turned to another local practitioner. Dr. Blaw used a special electronic machine (to be precise, an EAV machine, "electro-acupuncture according to Voll") that was supposed to diagnose food allergies. Greatly to Shirley's satisfaction, it gave her a long list of new foods that she and her daughter would have to avoid.

Even more exciting, the machine "diagnosed" sensitivity to electro-magnetic fields. This meant that Shirley could now blame her moods on electric power lines. While retaining all her dietary restrictions, she also installed reflective apparatus around all the beds in the house and purchased special crystals billed as being able to "neutralize electromagnetism."

I heard all this secondhand, from a mutual friend. There was nothing more I could do, so I tried to forget about it. But her daughter's fate haunted me. I wished I could help.

By chance, when I moved from Kansas City, Missouri, to Olympia Washington, Shirley moved, too. When Jane turned twelve, I began to notice her around town by herself, dressed all in black. She'd occasionally come up to me to chat, so I knew about it when at thirteen she started running away from home, sleeping on the streets, smoking cigarettes, and begging for food. She spent much of her fourteenth year in juvenile detention for petty thefts.

It was terrible to watch, but inwardly I was hopeful. Jane was trying to find her own life, trying to discover her own actual feelings rather than interpret her soul through the symbology of forbidden foods.

She called me a month or so after her seventeenth birthday. She was living with an aunt and going to junior college. "What did you think about all that crazy food stuff we used to talk about?" she asked. "I realized the other day that you never actually told us to eat weird. Did you believe in my mother's health food stuff or not?"

"I thought it was a bunch of crap," I said. "I still do."

She laughed. "Why didn't you say so?"

"You were a kid. What could I say? 'Your mom's out of her head'?"

"I guess not."

"I'm really sorry I couldn't do more. I felt terrible."

"Thanks . . . but what I really want to know is if I need to quit eating wheat again? Will I really die of migraine headaches? That's what my mother keeps telling me."

"You might get migraine headaches if you eat wheat," I said, "but you're not going to die from them. And what makes you think you're even going to get headaches anyway? You never had a migraine when you were a kid. They were your mother's migraines."

I could feel the smile coming through the phone line. "You mean I don't have to give up pizza?" she asked.

"Actually," I said, "you really don't." Then I launched into a favorite story of mine about a woman who *cured* herself by going on a beer and pizza diet (see Chapter 13).

For many people with migraines, eliminating a few allergenic foods might be just the ticket. Evidence suggests that migraine sufferers might be able to reduce the number and severity of headaches by leaving out chocolate, avocados, peanuts, and a couple of other foods (although a recent study found that chocolate had no effect). However, as always, we have to keep a sense of proportion. When we go overboard like Shirley, we may create an emotional illness that not only makes us crazy but can inflict considerable harm on a child as well.

As it happened, Jane did suffer occasional migraines. She came to see me professionally and asked, with trepidation, whether I'd reconsider having her eliminate allergenic foods. I shook my head emphatically no. Instead I recommended she take a pill for her headaches and entirely avoid thinking about food solutions. It would be decades, at least, before she'd have much chance of using food as a treatment for any illness without getting crazy over it again.

ORTHOREXIA AND ADDICTION

The Utne Reader titled its version of my initial orthorexia article "Confessions of a Health Food Junkie," and there's more to the concept than simply a funny title. Can one really develop an addiction to healthy food? The short answer is yes. It happens all the time, and it is one of the fundamental elements of orthorexia.

This may seem strange, as the term "addiction" connotes something bad for you, a substance like heroin or an activity like compulsive gambling. Yet positive experiences can become addictive as well. Workaholism is one classic example—we even praise workaholics for their addiction. Therapist Ellen Montague tells of another:

> *Although I've rock-climbed for many years, for one summer it became an addiction. I call it that because it had similar characteristics to other addictions. These include obsession, experiencing happiness only through the addiction, loss of other interests, secrecy, denial, defensiveness, and narrowing of my social circle.*
>
> *I exhibited all these traits that summer. I thought about rock climbing all the time (obsession); I wasn't happy unless I was climbing (only one way to be happy); I spent a lot of time when I wasn't climbing reading climbing books and looking at my climbing gear (narrowing of interests); I didn't tell others about any of this except maybe in a joking way (secrecy); and of course I didn't think I had a problem (denial). No one asked me about my climbing and how much time I spent on it, but if anyone had, I would have bristled (defensiveness). I certainly didn't spend much time with people unless they were climbers (narrowing of social circle). Luckily for me, something shifted on its own, and by the next summer I again had a healthy relationship with climbing.*
>
> *The same pieces that happened for me around rock climbing can happen about food. Neither of these addictions is likely to kill you. However, they do narrow your life.*

Orthorexia frequently shares all but one of the characteristics of addiction as well.

By definition an orthorexic is obsessed with food. For many orthorexics, eating food becomes the only way to feel happy. Narrowing of interests is a prime characteristic of any complex food theory such as macrobiotics, because nothing else in life seems so relevant and exciting as the food theory itself. Orthorexia intrinsically involves denial, since to an orthorexic the disease is a virtue. If you try to tell a follower of a food theory that he or she needs to loosen up, you'll instantly encounter defensiveness. Finally, orthorexia tends to narrow one's social circle down to those who follow a similar theory. The only glaring exception to this list is secrecy, or rather the lack of it. Orthorexics don't keep their fascination secret; they invariably talk about it with everyone in sight.

Not every orthorexic is addicted to health food. However, when obsession with healthy food begins to crowd out other concerns, when the thought of not eating such food fills us with dread and terror, when we will go to absurd lengths to obtain the food that we feel we need, the resemblance to more obvious forms of addiction begins to come clear.

Daniel was an adherent of macrobiotics (see Chapter 8 for more information on macrobiotics) and a health food addict. He was single, and had been for almost a decade. He was constantly in pursuit of relationships, but whenever one began, he soon found it stressful. By coincidence at that moment it would suddenly become extremely important to obtain some special Japanese dietary ingredient or to cut his vegetables with mathematical precision. These quests for dietary perfection would occupy so much of his time that the object of his affection would lose patience and go away, unable to compete with his primary relationship—the one with food. Then he'd be safe.

There is one way, however, in which health food addiction can be a positive force: when it replaces other, more dangerous addictions. According to some viewpoints, the essence of a good life involves "trading up" from one addiction to a healthier one. In this sense, it might be quite a good idea for someone addicted to drugs or alcohol to become interested in food. However, even in this interpretation addiction to healthy food needs to be transcended eventually.

As this book progresses, we will repeatedly return to the theme of addiction. Furthermore, as we shall see in Chapter 15, the paths out of orthorexia bear a distinct resemblance to twelve-step programs that have proven so uniquely successful in freeing people from chemical dependency.

Do you recognize yourself anywhere in this chapter? Do you suspect that your eating habits may be more of a problem than you want to admit? The next chapter will provide an informal test to determine whether you have orthorexia.

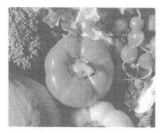

4.

Do You Have Orthorexia?

If you are a dietary zealot and enjoy spending every waking moment thinking about food, what you have is a life's mission, not an illness. But if you find yourself chafing against the restraints you've self-defined, if you've grown sick of obsessing over food, if the first chapters of this book have struck a chord, maybe it's time to think about your food habits as a problem rather than a virtue.

Here's a ten-question quiz to determine if you have orthorexia. If you answer yes to two or three of these questions, you have at least a touch of orthorexia. A score of four or more means that you are in trouble. And if all these statements apply to you, you really need help. You don't have a life—you have a menu!

THE ORTHOREXIA SELF-TEST

Give yourself a point for each "yes" answer.

1. Do you spend more than three hours a day thinking about healthy food? (For four hours, give yourself two points.)

The time measurement here includes cooking, shopping, reading about your diet, discussing (or evangelizing) it with friends, and joining Internet chat groups on the subject. Three hours a day is too much to think about healthy food.

Life is meant for joy, love, passion, and accomplishment. Absorption with righteous food seldom produces any of these things, and if you find yourself regularly joyous about zucchini, in love with raw-grain pizza, passionate about amaranth, or proud of your ability to eat nothing but brown rice, your priorities are out of place. Remember, life is too short to be spent thinking about how healthy or unhealthy your diet is.

2. Do you plan tomorrow's food today?

Orthorexics tend to dwell on upcoming menus. "Today I will eat steamed broccoli, while tomorrow I will boil Swiss chard. The day after that I think I'll make brown rice with adzuki beans." If you get a thrill of pleasure from contemplating a healthy menu the day after tomorrow, something is wrong with your focus.

3. Do you care more about the virtue of what you eat than the pleasure you receive from eating it?

It's one thing to love to eat, but for an orthorexic it isn't the food itself; it's the idea of the food. You can pump yourself up so giddily with pride that you don't even taste it going down.

On several Web sites devoted to eating, correspondents have objected to the very notion of orthorexia on the grounds that animals spend most of *their* day thinking about eating. Why shouldn't people do so as well?

But an animal's passion for food is related to hunger and survival. In orthorexia, hunger itself is secondary. It's the meaning of food that attracts, and it is precisely the excessive meaning attached to food that makes orthorexia a disorder.

4. Have you found that as the quality of your diet has increased, the quality of your life has correspondingly diminished?

The problem with orthorexia is that healthy food doesn't feed your soul. Living with passion feeds your soul. If you spend too much energy on what you put into your mouth, pretty soon the meaning will drain out of the rest of your life.

Be honest with yourself. Which do you think really matters more: spending two hours with your child or devoting that two hours to cooking a macrobiotic meal? Listening to your friend or thoughtfully savoring the taste of an orange? Volunteering in your community or fasting every Friday?

5. Do you keep getting stricter with yourself?

Like other addictions, orthorexia tends to escalate, demanding increasing vigilance as time passes. The diet of yesterday isn't pure enough for tomorrow. Over time the rules governing healthy eating get more rigid. And if you are an orthorexic, you get a grim pleasure from this.

For example, while macrobiotic diet considers brown rice, vegetables, and tofu healthy (as indeed they are), adherents feel that they are even more virtuous if they eat only brown rice. Similarly, raw-foodists may graduate to fruitarianism (eating only fruit) and then breatharianism (living on air only). Those who are afraid of allergenic foods tend to progressively eliminate everything but turkey and white rice. (See Chapters 6 and 7 for more information on these food theories.)

It is all a miserly illusion. After a certain point of reasonable dietary improvements, neither happiness nor health comes from increasing strictness.

6. Do you sacrifice experiences you once enjoyed to eat the food you believe is right?

Because of its confused scale of values, orthorexia leads to a crazy allocation of interest. Have you fallen into this trap? Will you turn down an invitation to eat at a friend's house because the food there isn't healthy enough for you? Do you find that obsessive thoughts of healthy food occupy your mind while you watch your child perform a play at school? Would you, like Claire, avoid marriage with someone you really think you could love just because he eats the wrong food?

7. Do you feel an increased sense of self-esteem when you are eating healthy food? Do you look down on others who don't?

One of the seductive aspects of orthorexia is that it allows one to feel superior to other people. After all, healthy eating is everywhere extolled. Orthorexia seems to be right up there with good work habits and a clean life. In this, orthorexia has an aspect that can make it harder to shake than other eating disorders: While anorexics and bulimics feel ashamed of their habits, orthorexics strut with pride. "Look at those degenerates," the mind says of everyone else, "hopelessly addicted to junk."

This pride is insidious. Because orthorexics revel in their disease, they cannot easily arrive at the need to change. When they've bottomed out, they think they've reached the summit.

In fact, orthorexia is a vice, not a virtue, and pride in it is a corrosive form of self-deception (not to mention the universal fact that feeling superior to others is a sick way to live). As with alcoholism (or, even more to the point in this case, workaholism), the first step is to admit to yourself that you have a problem.

8. Do you feel guilt or self-loathing when you stray from your diet?

If you are an orthorexic, you feel guilt and shame when you eat foods that don't fit the anointed diet. Your sense of self-esteem is so linked to what you eat that tasting a morsel of forbidden food feels like a sin. The only way to regain self-respect is to recommit yourself to ever-stricter eating, to despise yourself when you stray from the path of food righteousness.

Of course, there are times in life when it is worthwhile feeling ashamed. We all often fail to reach the mark and need to let ourselves feel the disappointment. When I've lost my temper at a child, betrayed a secret, insulted a friend behind his back, I've committed an actual error worthy of actual guilt.

But eating pizza is fairly low on the scale of vital moral lapses. No one on her deathbed looks back and says, "I am filled with regret that I ate too much ice cream and not enough kale."

9. Does your diet socially isolate you?

Once you've reached a certain point, the rigidity demanded by orthorexia makes it truly difficult for you to eat anywhere but at home. Most restaurants don't serve the right foods, and even when they do, you won't trust that it will be prepared correctly. Even your friends inexplicably fail to cater to your personal preferences (or, as you see it, they willfully choose to ignore the one right way of eating).

You have very limited choices when it comes to social gatherings.

You can go and refuse to eat. Once I slowly sliced and ate (with feigned gusto) a single orange while everyone else consumed a five-course homemade feast. Another approach is to order your hosts to prepare food according to your standards (but they will inevitably fail).

The more common strategy is to bring your own food in separate containers and chew it slowly, looking virtuous and soulful while everyone else gulps down garbage. Or, like a solitary alcoholic, you can decline the invitation and dine in the loneliness and comfort of your own home.

Orthorexia makes it difficult to keep friends. Your friends have to eat what you eat or feel the sting of your condemnation. You are not a lot of fun to be friends with anymore.

10. When you are eating the way you are supposed to, do you feel a peaceful sense of total control?

Life is complicated, unpredictable, and often scary. It is not always possible to control your life, but you can control what you eat. A heavy-handed domination over what goes onto your fork or spoon can create the comfortable illusion that your life is no longer in danger of veering from the plan.

But no matter what you eat, life takes its own turns. Like an alcoholic nursing a bottle, you can stare at your plate all you want, but the world still goes on outside your grasp. Your dominion over the world of food cuts little cake with the Fates.

If you just racked up enough points to diagnose orthorexia, it's time to disinfect your mind. Before turning to the general methods for gaining freedom from health food bondage, I need to talk about what causes orthorexia. Next I'll dissect a few famous dietary theories, with the intention of helping you stop treating their recommendations as gospel truth. Finally I'll turn to subject of breaking free, in Section 3.

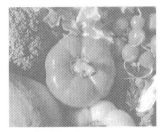

5.

Hidden Causes
of Orthorexia

There are many legitimate reasons to seek out a healthier diet. Perhaps a friend or relative has died at a young age from heart disease, and your physician tells you you're at risk yourself. Or maybe you suffer from symptoms that conventional medicine cannot address, and a dietary theory sounds like a promising option for you. Many people just feel less than well and hope that by adopting a different way of eating they can increase their energy level and sense of well-being. These are all good and sensible reasons to change your diet, and none of them necessarily leads to orthorexia.

However, food is a highly charged topic. For most of us it is mixed up with love, a famous complication that has been widely discussed in the context of gaining weight. In orthorexia there are frequently other forces that take over, too, hidden causes that juice up the appeal of diet and make extremism the most natural course.

This chapter seeks to bring those hidden causes into the light.

WARREN'S STORY

How many times have you watched a friend live through a story like the following?

At about age thirty, Warren had a cancer scare. It started with a bad cold, and along with sneezing, coughing, and a sore throat, the lymph glands in his neck swelled up. This last symptom made him particularly nervous, and he couldn't stop fingering his glands, pushing on them, checking to see if they had shrunk or grown since the last time he'd touched them, five minutes before.

Within the usual week's period, the rest of his cold symptoms had disappeared, but the swollen glands remained, and they remained quite sore (if only from all the self-examination). Warren's anxiety continued to grow, because, as he explained to me, his mother had died from lymphatic cancer. He was obsessed with the notion that he might have it, too. He knew it wasn't logical—his mother had died at eighty-two, and her lymph-gland swelling had not begun with a cold—but he couldn't get it out of his mind.

The standard medical response in such situations is to wait a month and see if the glands don't shrink back to normal. I suggested this, resisting his impassioned desire to get a biopsy right then and there. He called me again in two weeks and showed up one month to the day after the last visit.

His neck was red from being rubbed, but his lymph glands seemed smaller to me. I wanted to give it a few more weeks. However, under the duress of his insistence, I sent him to a surgeon, who, equally under duress, agreed to a biopsy. It came back negative. The most likely diagnosis was simply an exaggerated response to a cold, and the glands would eventually go back to normal.

Warren was reassured for a few days, but then his imagination got back to work. He decided that a cancer was still brewing, only one too small as yet for us to detect. He started reading furiously about healing diets, and he finally decided that what he needed to do was "detoxify" himself. This term comes from traditional naturopathy (see Chapter 7) and involves various methods thought to purify the body. The particular form of the method he chose involved eating mostly raw foods, along with taking up fasting, colonics, and various herbs and supplements.

After about a month he felt he had achieved success, because his lymph nodes had returned to normal size. I carefully refrained from annoying him by pointing out that this was what usually happened on its own. He also felt energized, "cleaned out," and pure. What's more, his anxiety over developing cancer had disappeared, because he was sure that with his new diet all risk of getting sick had disappeared. Again I couldn't see any reason to mention that I disagreed.

He continued on his raw foods diet for another year, and even gave public and private lectures on it. (His friends and relatives were the victims of the private lectures.) But at the end of the year he fell ill with mononucleosis and stayed bedridden for six months. This gave him plenty of time to read, and when he finally came out of bed, he was a fanatical follower of macrobiotics, a dietary approach that bans all raw foods.

UNDER THE SURFACE: THE SEARCH FOR TOTAL SAFETY

At one level Warren was just looking for a way to improve his health. He decided, based on his reading, that first one diet and then another might be the best way of getting healthier. Even if I might be less impressed than he by the validity of the theories behind these diets, I certainly grant him the right to make whatever health decisions seem most logical to him. We all make our decisions based on what seems true, and it is absolutely right to do so.

But was this everything to the story? Did Warren have any other motivations behind a rational search for improved health?

I think it's pretty obvious that he did. It's not hard to see that many of Warren's actions were driven by fear rather than by choice. He was terrified and a bit of a hypochondriac, and he chose the path of extreme diets in order to allay his fears. He hoped to adopt a path that would *remove all health risk.*

Unfortunately, it's impossible to reduce to zero the risk of illness or accident. So long as you are a member of a mortal species—a membership that it is difficult to alter—you are susceptible to unpredictable illnesses and other health risks. You can reduce those risks by being careful, but you can't make them go away altogether. Even people with the healthiest possible diets get sick sometimes, even badly so, and eventually we all die. There's a great deal of chance involved along the way, combined with numerous factors that diet cannot overcome.

Of course, it is perfectly advisable to take steps to reduce your chance of illness. I am greatly in favor of a low-fat, semivegetarian or vegetarian diet, accompanied by healthy lifestyle habits and regular exercise. But Warren went wrong, in my opinion, and passed from healthy choices to orthorexia, when he tried to reduce his risk to zero.

Whenever we try to make ourselves completely safe, we are engaged in a fantasy, and the mental force required to carry out this feat of make-believe drives us a little crazy. When it comes to food, such game-playing leads to orthorexia. We throw all the weight of our fears into a diet that we unrealistically imagine will make us completely safe. It's analogous to marrying someone in the belief that all your happiness will come from that person. It's incorrect, impossible, wrongheaded, and fundamentally doomed to fail. By pretending that a diet will make you completely safe, you start on a path of illusion that builds over time.

THE HIDDEN CAUSES OF ORTHOREXIA

Orthorexia usually has at least one hidden cause, a mythical belief that is deeply attractive but, unfortunately, untrue. I call Warren's fantasy the Illusion of Total Safety. It's closely allied to another common desire underlying orthorexia, the Desire for Complete Control. But these aren't the only hidden agendas of orthorexia. Here are the most important:

- Illusion of Total Safety
- Desire for Complete Control
- Covert Conformity
- Searching for Spirituality in the Kitchen
- Food Puritanism
- Creating an Identity
- Fear of Other People

Illusion of Total Safety
As I described earlier, the Illusion of Total Safety allows us to pretend that we can forever ward off illness. We can't control the pollution in the air we breathe, the many potentially toxic chemicals we absorb through the skin, the genes we were born with, the behavior

of drunken drivers, or the steady creep, creep of aging. However, we can grab with extra desperation the one thing we can control and that might keep us healthy—eating.

To a certain extent it is true. By eating properly (along with exercising regularly and developing a healthy support system) we can increase, on average, our life span and reduce, on average, the risk of developing a host of nasty illnesses.

However, the catch is "on average." We don't live our lives statistically; we are each a sample of one. Furthermore, no matter what we do, aging and death will catch up with us.

You might ask, What's the problem with pretending you are going to live forever? Why not avoid facing these big, ugly realities? Unfortunately, there's a huge cost to this pretense. By pretending you can remove all risks, you lose the ability to grow from facing those risks.

At some point in our lives (usually considerably past the teenage years!), we ordinarily discover that we are mortal, that the clock is ticking away and our interval of life is going to end someday. When faced directly, this terrifying experience becomes a source of growth toward maturity. It helps us to sort out our priorities, to pay attention to what really matters, perhaps to value the people in our lives more now that we know we won't be knowing them forever. And we prune through the options in our lives to settle on what matters most.

But if we use food as a diversion from mortality, or a screen to pretend that it doesn't exist, we don't take this step. We continue to live with an adolescent mind, imagining that life will go on forever. This is not as great a harm as dying from anorexia, but it is still a huge loss. For the truth is that we don't live very long on earth, and until we come to terms with this fact, we don't really live at all. When we use food to create an illusion of perfect safety, it robs us of the chance to take one of the greatest growth steps of adult life.

Consider Audrey, a seventy-five-year-old woman who had achieved this age without ever acknowledging that her life span was less than infinite. She was a great frequenter of health food stores and a popper of pills, her skin was a bit orange from all the carrot juice she tossed down the way other people toss down sodas, and she was always going off for an enema, sauna, or acupuncture treatment (the last provided by me).

Most of Audrey's life revolved around her diet. She followed no one program in particular but managed to gather together suggestions from Edgar Cayce, Gaylord Hauser, and Jethro Kloss to create an impressively complex regimen that involved twelve meals a day, each consisting of only a single food. In addition, she took perhaps eighty food supplements or herbal pills a day and consumed heroic quantities of wheat germ, royal jelly, kelp, blue-green algae, and apple cider vinegar.

I knew Audrey for more than a year before I found out she had grandchildren. They lived in the same town, and she did take care of them occasionally, but not too often, as they "get awfully impatient while I'm preparing my meals, and they also make me lose count of my pills."

She did get out every day, but only to either exercise, buy food, or get her enema, sauna, or acupuncture treatment. Her exercising consisted of fast walking around a local track, eight turns a day, for four miles, rain or shine. Excellent exercise, but she did it alone, and so far as I could tell, she didn't enjoy being outdoors. It was just a cold-blooded attempt at life extension, a carefully reasoned and deliberate stress upon the heart for health's sake only.

Audrey seemed to me like someone who was forever preparing for a race, building herself up for some future event that justified so much time spent in the present. But the race was against death; her preparation would never have an end, until she lost. In the meantime she wasn't living. She was so concerned with being safe that she forgot what she was staying safe *for,* so concerned with life extension that she had forgotten to live.

I tried for two years to get her to consider doing something in her life other than trying to extend it, but I got nowhere. It was obvious that she was desperately afraid of dying. However, instead of facing up to this, she sublimated it all into dietary complexities. I couldn't find a single point of contact. I wished that one of the authors she trusted so much had included a note of balance, a recommendation to consider other values than length of life.

It was mortality itself that finally helped Audrey let go of the Illusion of Total Safety. A sudden stroke paralyzed half her body. When I visited her at the hospital, I saw the change immediately. The screen of food was gone. She looked right at me, and along with terror her eyes showed a vitality of feeling I'd never seen there before.

When she finally got out of the hospital, Audrey turned her life around in short order. She joined a religious group, one of whose major tenets was to face death honestly. She started calling up people who really mattered to her and told them so. An old but long-estranged friend came out to visit, and from what I heard from Audrey, they reconciled beautifully. Finally she realized that she might have very little time left to see her grandchildren, and she tried as best she could with her crippled body to get to know them better.

How did she eat during this time? Probably better than 95 percent of Americans, but she no longer thought about it at all. When life itself reclaimed its rightful place in her life, food receded.

Desire for Complete Control

Closely related to the quest for absolute safety through food is the Desire for Complete Control. In this case it is not just illness that you try to overcome through food, it's all the unpredictability of life.

Life does have a way of confounding our expectations. Just when you think it is going to zag, it zigs instead. Really, this is the most interesting part of life; it's what makes real existence better than a video game. But it's scary. Everything *seems* under control, and then along comes a person, an event, an act of nature that turns it all upside down. We never tire of trying to manage life to keep ourselves and those we love secure, but it never quite works out. An illness comes from nowhere, a teenager attempts suicide, a flood washes out the basement, or a semi runs you off the road.

There's no getting around it. Even money won't help. There's nothing we can do to get control of life, not really, beyond taking sensible precautions. And strangely, the more we control our lives, the less satisfying they are. The true interest in being alive comes from its very unpredictability, the way life is alive rather than a movie.

In *A Grief Observed*, C. S. Lewis touches on this issue when writing about the death of his wife, Joy. One of his biggest sources of grief was a subtle one: After a few months he realized that she was already becoming a static memory. In real life she had been unpredictable, surprising, entirely herself. Now she was turning into a fixed portrait, a perfect woman who aroused marvelous memories but never overturned his habits just by being herself. Lewis realized that he liked it when she upset his applecart; the way her memory rapidly turned her into a porcelain doll made his heart ache.

For Lewis this became clear only after Joy died. Sometimes while we are in a relationship we actually wish our partner would be a fixed and predictable object. We are annoyed by those quirks, oddities, and rough edges. However, if someone we loved really were to stay within the bounds of our expectations, we would rapidly become bored and the relationship sterile. It would be like marrying yourself. Wanting a relationship to stay within fixed bounds is actually not wanting a relationship at all.

It's the same with every other part of life. Wanting life to stay within its limits and never to penetrate, by its surprising changes, the boundaries we have set for ourselves is like asking life not be life; it is like choosing *The Truman Show* over stepping out of the dome.

In orthorexia, we try to make life safe by focusing on one easily controlled part of it: food. In order to avoid awareness of the chaos of existence, we pick one area over which we can be absolute lord and master, and that is the embarrassingly self-involved one of diet.

Of all food theories, macrobiotics (see Chapter 8) perhaps most completely satisfies the craving for a feeling of control. This dietary philosophy involves so many rules and attaches such grand significance to the small details of eating that it is easy to come to believe that by managing your diet properly, life will inevitably all fall into place. As one patient, Sarah, said to me, "So long as I keep the yin and the yang of my body balanced, everything in my life outside will stay in balance, too. Work, relationships, even so-called chance events are actually under the influence of my own inner balance."

Unfortunately, two weeks after she'd told me this, Sarah's mobile home was washed away in a flood, and with it all her sense of peaceful equilibrium. Life doesn't really modify its flow to match our diet. To think it does is an illusion.

However, it's a persistent and seductive illusion. Turning to a food theory feels so comforting when life is getting weird. There is so much peace in properly arranging the vegetables and rice on your plate, such a sense of safety in complying with all the dietary rules. I followed macrobiotics myself at one time, and I vividly remember how the anxiety and distress of going to medical school would melt away, all the uncertainty over the stress and time pressure would dissolve, all the feeling that my life was controlled by unpredictable forces outside my control would vanish as I contemplated the world of my dinner plate, where I was king.

As with so many stories of my own orthorexia, it is embarrassing even to recall this state of mind. I was like a heroin addict who retreats from real-life problems into an opiate daze where everything is fine. Everything was fine on my plate. Oh, certainly, I had some problems—the carrots weren't sliced just right, and I wasn't able to build up the fortitude to eat nothing but long-grain brown rice. Those little problems were part of how the escape worked; they took my energy and gave me the illusion of overcoming real difficulties. It was such a safe little world.

Then into my world of carefully ordered food perfection came a life-threatening illness. Food remedies didn't work. My sense of complete control over life was flooded away by the evident power of life to expel me if it so chose. I couldn't play house with my dietary rules; real life was in charge.

And looking back, I can hardly wish I had stayed in my glass cage, my imaginary world of dietary perfection. It has been better to live life as a sometimes dizzy and overwhelmed participant rather than to feel safe in an imaginary world of perfect control. It's much more satisfying to forget the pretense of controlling things and decide to bounce up and down as life careens along, to improvise and respond spontaneously, to accept and appreciate life's surprises. Also, once we face the reality of death, it stops popping up like a monster from under the bed; like other demons, death is least scary when most directly faced. Trying to pretend it away only gives it greater power.

Covert Conformity

Therapist Ellen Montague uses the expression "Covert Conformity" to describe a very common hidden agenda behind orthorexia, especially among women. It refers to the way a dietary theory can allow women to seek the culturally accepted norms of beauty without admitting it to themselves. Simply put, vegans, raw-foodists, and macrobiotic followers are usually very thin. It's a kind of side effect of the diet. If you follow one of these theories, you can "accidentally" live up to the Barbie image without admitting you believe in doing so.

> *Montague writes: I first became vegetarian at age twenty for ethical reasons only. Issues of weight or attractiveness didn't come into it. However, over time I noticed that my peers who ate a standard American diet were gaining weight while I was staying thin. I gradually started making the connection that vegetarians were thinner people. I didn't think I had any issues with weight myself, but I did notice this.*
>
> *Then, as I aged, I slowly began to gain weight. Twenty years after high school I found that I'd gained twenty-five pounds. Subtly,*

almost imperceptibly, I began to become interested in my weight.
But I wouldn't have admitted it to anyone, least of all to myself.

In 1991, I stopped consuming milk products to try to cure some
other health problems. During the process, I lost ten pounds. There
are fattening non-dairy desserts, I suppose, but you won't find them
on the table at potlucks. I'd eat my fruit salad while everyone else
had cheesecake. I wasn't trying to lose weight, mind you. I don't do
weight-loss diets. I was just trying to stay healthy. But did I mind
that I was now thinner?

I stayed away from milk products for many years. The ostensible
reason was that I felt healthier. However, a hidden fear played into
that decision: the fear that I would gain the ten pounds back again.
Of course, I didn't present this as my main reason for staying away
from milk products. I cloaked the avoidance in much more politi-
cally correct terms. "I'm feeling healthier," I'd tell myself and others.
"I don't get as many colds. I'm eating lower on the food chain, and
anyway it's more spiritually advanced."

Eventually, I did start eating milk products again, and, just as I
feared, those ten pounds came back. (All you who are going to stop
eating milk products because of this last paragraph, you know who
you are.)

It took me a long time to admit this hidden agenda to myself.
Now it seems obvious. Can you imagine a new way of eating that
would have a chapter titled "Eat this way and you'll be much
healthier, and also gain a lot of weight." No, of course not. It
wouldn't sell, not even to men.

It's so hard to avoid the conditioning around weight, the impos-
sible standards that women, in particular, are supposed to achieve. I
have yet to meet a woman who is satisfied with her body's current

shape. However, in alternative circles, we don't talk about weight, but rather about fitness. "Oh, I'm so out of shape," we say.

So now it's clear that a large piece of my own orthorexia has been about trying to conform to standards of attractiveness while not admitting it. On the surface, I didn't want to try to look like a model. I spent years of my life avoiding that whole compulsion, because I believed (and still believe) that those norms of beauty are oppressive, are a function of sick things about our society, and so on. And yet inside, I secretly wanted to feel attractive. Hence, any dietary theory that might help me lose weight made my ears perk up.

Fasting, too. I told my friends that I fasted annually to clean out my system. I do believe this. But I also secretly believed that if I fasted I would lose weight. I also hoped it would reset my metabolism, so I wouldn't gain weight again as quickly.

As I've started to show signs of aging (wrinkles, gray hair), I've become even more obsessed with my weight. I can't make the wrinkles go away, but I can get thinner.

At least now I can admit it to myself. And maybe, by being honest, I can change the pattern. Because I don't want to be obsessed either with food or my weight. It's no way to live.

Searching for Spirituality in the Kitchen

A completely different force behind orthorexia is the search for spirituality. Humans have found ways to seek God in churches, mosques, temples, mountain shrines, desert retreats, and the full-voiced joys of great musical choirs. Perhaps it shouldn't be surprising, then, when people have tried to find God in the kitchen. This "kitchen spirituality" can cause some of the severest forms of orthorexia.

Macrobiotics *is* actually a religion, a form of Taoism transferred to food. (To be precise, it parallels religious Taoism, a heavily ritualized system that in many ways is precisely the opposite of the free-flowing worldview of the *Tao Te Ching*.) When you practice macrobiotics, you focus extreme care on such issues as just precisely how you slice your carrots, and make calculations regarding the spiritual balance of your food reminiscent of a chemistry class. You analyze your food based on local climate, the season of the year, daily weather, and numerous other aspects of your personal life. The goal is to eat in precisely balanced harmony with your environment and thereby promote unity of mind, body, and soul. A lofty and noble goal, no doubt, but perhaps it is a bit misplaced when applied to food.

Raw-foodism, another dietary sect, doesn't seek balance. Rather, it finds spirituality by cultivating in followers an angelic state while living on earth. Transparency, lightness, and glowing clarity are the goal, along with a deep appreciation of the fundamental gifts of nature. "Fruit is love," says Jeremy Safron, the owner of Raw Experience, a raw foods restaurant in San Francisco. He means that trees give up their fruit voluntarily, hoping that it will be eaten, as a kind of free gift to the world. Unlike other foods, fruit doesn't run away from you. The trees want you to eat it. By doing so, you become one with the giving spirit of the world.

There's certainly something beautifully innocent, if absurd, about the most extreme of raw foods followers. "I'm like the messiah to bring in the new world," says Juliano, the founder of Raw Experience. Somehow I rather doubt that most people on earth would really want a messianic aura orbiting around their raw wheat pizzas.

Like other religions, kitchen spirituality evangelizes. Most followers of food theories think everyone else should join them in their particular obsession. Macrobiotics and raw foods theory explicitly state a goal of converting everyone to their respective (and in many ways opposite) creeds; their diets will end war, disease, famine, and everything else that's bad in the world.

Other eating theories do not make converting others part of the catechism, but it tends to follow anyway from the universal human tendency to think that what's true for me is true for everyone else. Vegans notoriously lay guilt trips on anyone who eats meat. And people with food allergies believe that anyone who comes down with a cold shares their personal sensitivities.

There's nothing fundamentally wrong with finding God in food. Spiritual seekers have found God everywhere and anywhere. But the problem with kitchen spirituality is that it gets stuck on food. It contracts the soul rather than expands it; it adjusts the spirit to the confines of an orange instead of spreading it into the sky.

True, gratitude for one's meal is a traditional component of spirituality. However, one blesses a meal because it is a blessing to have anything to eat at all. When you start blessing the entrée because it contains stir-fried vegetables cosmically balanced to the right yin and yang or the fruit salad because the fruit is cut raw so recently it seems to glow with etheric force, you have made the food itself a deity, not thanked the deity behind the food.

If healthy eating were so spiritual, wouldn't you expect that religions would make it a central tenet? Certainly, religions have their food restrictions, but they don't elevate eating to the same level as, say, love, morality, devotion, and good works. Orthorexics think that food and spirituality are identical, but great spiritual figures do not.

I saw this dichotomy back in the late seventies, while staying at a house where the Karmapa was visiting. The Karmapa is one of the major spiritual leaders of the Tibetan people. Unlike the Dalai Lama, who plays more of a secular role, the Karmapa's place in Tibetan culture is purely spiritual. He is (or rather was, as the Karmapa of this story has since died and the identification of his successor remains in dispute) considered a great master of meditation and a fount of spiritual wisdom.

I was visiting an old friend who lived in a Tibetan Buddhist center in Santa Cruz, California, during the time of the Karmapa's visit. It was the occasion of much anxiety, excitement, and orthorexic planning. My friend John had supervised the construction of an appropriate throne for the evening's presentation, and many other enthusiastic California Buddhists had performed similar feats of amateur accomplishment. The house was rich with roses and the kitchen well stocked with the nutritious and healthful delicacies everyone imagined the great teacher would prefer to eat.

The night before the Karmapa's arrival, a protocol expert from San Francisco had come down to advise us on proper deportment. Much of her advice was expected: John was to greet the Karmapa at the driveway with a bouquet of burning incense, other lamas would station themselves about the entrance of the house and blow Tibetan horns, no alcohol was permitted in the house, and so forth. One feature of the ritual was, however, a bit troubling: Protocol, it turned out, demanded that all those in the presence of the Karmapa keep their heads down below the level of his. Considering that he was much shorter than an average American, this presented quite a prospect of sore backs and heads.

When we asked the expert about the food we had picked out for the Karmapa, she simply smiled, a response we mistakenly took for approval.

The Karmapa arrived precisely on schedule the next morning,

ten minutes after another black Mercedes that disgorged the advance guard of lamas with horns. As the Karmapa emerged from his Mercedes, the lamas blasted an eerie instrumental greeting that brought the rest of the neighborhood to their windows, doors, and balconies. He walked slowly up the driveway and acknowledged John and the burning incense.

The Karmapa exuded a regal aura, and his slight lurch and stiffness of face caused by advanced brain cancer only made him appear more imposing. At his side, however, came a disreputable-looking Tibetan who also lurched slightly as he walked, but in a different, looser sort of way. His bedraggled hair hung down over a multilayered motley of brightly colored but dirty Tibetan vests and shirts. He carried a bottle in his left hand and swigged it as he came in the door. It was impossible to miss the scent of alcohol, but as the whispered word came around, we discovered that he was the Karmapa's childhood friend, Ludra, and entitled to break the rules.

We offered the Karmapa a feast of whole-grain sandwiches with garbanzo bean spread, a salad made of six varieties of organically grown lettuce, all to be washed down with freshly pressed carrot juice, but to our great surprise he waved it away. The interpreter explained that he wanted to go to the amusement park before eating.

Although confused by this request, we complied, and in company with the two black Mercedeses we drove to the Santa Cruz boardwalk. Our ensemble made a peculiar picture, I'm sure—the Karmapa in the lead in his long robes, walking stiffly but with dignity; beside him, his drunken childhood friend; to the side, robed lamas; and behind, a troop of American Buddhists, bent over steeply. We were going toward "Mr. Toad's Wild Ride," an amusement the Karmapa had heard about in advance and apparently wanted to sample.

The ride was a bumper-car arena. It created an immediate problem, because to all the Buddhists, bumping the Karmapa would have been a sacrilegious act. The Karmapa drove about wildly, and all the rest of us had to steer like madmen to avoid striking him. We could ram each other, however, as much as we wanted, and the resulting pileup left us all laughing hilariously and relaxed.

Until the subject of food returned. The Karmapa made an announcement after the ride that shook the faith of many of his American followers and nearly caused some of them to turn away from Buddhism entirely. For how could a Buddhist do such a thing? This man, this Karmapa, believed to be an embodiment of wisdom and a fount of understanding, capable of miracles on earth and of consciously reincarnating after death, this divine figure asked to go to McDonald's. It appeared that he was inordinately fond of Big Macs.

Had he recommended robbing a bank I don't think the grumbling and discontent would have been much louder. My memory is tinged with humor, but at the time it didn't seem funny at all. How could he suggest this? How could he want it?

"No wonder he has cancer," whispered a young woman who I knew was a vegan. "Maybe his cancer has made him a little crazy?" another offered by way of defense. "Do we have to eat with him?" another asked, quite forgetting the immense spiritual benefit that was supposed to accrue from time spent with the Karmapa.

But Tibetan Buddhism does not ever make a point of enjoining healthy eating. The native diet, after all, is rich with yak fat. The religion emphasizes meditation, compassion, and self-discipline, not health food. The association between Buddhist spiritual advancement and good diet was an American fabrication, nowhere suggested except in the minds of the Karmapa's orthorexic followers, who thought that their obsession was the natural obsession of all good and right-thinking people. It simply isn't true. Spirituality and food are not one and the same; kitchen spirituality is an aberration.

Food Puritanism

A completely different semireligious motivation can underlie orthorexia: the desire for self-deprivation. I call this "food puritanism." It is extremely common in the alternative medicine world, undertaken with a naïve enthusiasm that fails entirely to recognize what is going on.

From the time of the execution of King Charles I to the Restoration of 1660, the Puritans ruled England. Theaters were closed, dancing and singing restricted, and bearbaiting was forbidden (it was commonly said), not because of the pain it caused the bear but because of the pleasure it caused the watchers. It was a time of severity in which all pleasures, if not found strictly wholesome, were looked upon as evil.

The impulse to deny what is spontaneously pleasurable has a long history throughout the world. Its most extreme form, asceticism, was equally popular in Europe, India, and Japan for millennia. The hair shirt of the medieval monk, the self-starvation of the Indian *sadhu*, the indifference to pleasures of the Roman stoics—it all comes from the same impulse: to deny the desires of the flesh in order to focus on what really matters.

Few people today, even the most religious, subscribe to the doctrines of asceticism. Quite the contrary, our culture believes that a certain spontaneity, a certain wholeness of life is normal, healthy, and admirable. Nonetheless, we still admire those who live ascetically: Gandhi and Mother Teresa being two figures who come to mind. But we don't require it. When Nelson Mandela remarried at the age of eighty, we considered it a sign of the largeness of his being. In fact, if a person today were to live his life so seriously that he found all enjoyments a distraction, we would look at him as strange, and distrust him. This, indeed, was the reaction to Supreme Court Justice David Souter, when it was found that he lived alone and reused his yogurt containers.

In the field of natural health, however, puritanism is alive and well. I recently edited a series of books on alternative medicine, most of which were written by physicians involved with natural medicine. I was surprised to find how often I ran across paragraphs somewhat like the following parody:

> *All of us know what we need to do to achieve optimum health. But do we really follow the rules of healthy living? Nooo. Think about it. How often have you decided to drink a cup of coffee, regardless of its terrible consequences for your health, or indulged yourself in a chocolate bar full of unhealthy oils and indigestible cooked nuts? No wonder we get sick so often. Cancer, heart disease, frequent colds, allergies, and the breakdown of the immune system can all be traced to our degenerate habit of living to eat rather than eating to live.*
>
> *When you let your appetite for instant gratification guide your decisions and ignore what you know about what is good for you, it should be no surprise when you get sick. But do we learn? Too often not. Too often we eat for pleasure rather than for health, with all the predictable consequences.*

Admonitions like these would make Puritans sing hallelujahs in their graves. Such writing assumes that the enjoyment of eating is a guilty vice, tending toward the evil of disease. This assumption, taken as indisputable, maintains that there really is no reason to eat other than to maximize health, that any other motivation is shameful.

But what if you like drinking coffee? The reality is that there is no real evidence that coffee is harmful for you. Granted, it's probably not particularly healthy for you, unlike soybeans, and it may make you feel funny when the caffeine wears off. But if you like coffee, why not drink it in moderation? Where does the natural medicine doctor come off shaming you for enjoying your java?

Not only are chocolate, caffeine, and most other health vices probably harmless if taken in moderation, who says in the first place that the only purpose of eating is pure health? We don't just eat to live. We eat for pleasure. It is purely a puritan impulse to believe that pleasure is suspect.

Not that I haven't participated in shaming my patients over what they eat. While conventional doctors like to say, "It must be all in your head," we alternative doctors find plenty of ways to blame our patients. One of the most common is to pick at the patient's diet. "You mean you still have headaches? Now, confess, did you have any chocolate since I last saw you?"

"Yes," the patient meekly replies. "I did have one Hershey's Kiss."

I make a face, shake my head, and then launch into my speech.

"Well, no wonder, then. Didn't I tell you that for the first forty years you will have to strictly avoid all sugar and chocolate, not to mention caffeine, alcohol, salt, cheese, meat, milk, butter, fat, pepper, pasta, soy sauce, and artificial sweeteners? If you persist in being such a greedy, undisciplined, slovenly car wreck of a human being, when you get sick I want you to feel very, very guilty. You are a bad patient. I don't know if you will ever get better."

Okay, I'm exaggerating. We alternative doctors aren't actually that mean. But we do tend to set up a nearly impossible health regimen and then use it to avoid any sense of responsibility if the patient does not get well on schedule.

But who are we to decide that a person should not make a choice to indulge in unhealthy foods, as a matter of choice? It really is a choice, not in the sense of "You chose to do this, so no wonder you are sick," but rather "It appears to be healthier to eat X, but it's up to you to decide what is most important to you: the highest statistical probability of living a long time or enjoying eating Y."

When I was a child, a physician of mine decided I was allergic to wheat and milk. Perhaps this was true, perhaps it wasn't, but the upshot was that for me wheat and milk had become evil foods. If I ate ice cream, cake, a sandwich, or a cookie, I had "cheated."

To my mother's credit, she suggested that I "cheat" from time to time, even if it did make me sick. "It's worth it to have fun at a birthday party," she would say, "even if it does give you a little asthma." I remembered this for some time before forgetting it in my later descent into full-fledged orthorexia.

Like other extreme diets, food allergy theory tends to escalate, until practically no food is legal. The orthorexic takes a peculiarly cheerful attitude toward this self-denial, reacting with a gloomy pleasure upon reading a label and finding, as the nineteenth ingredient, a food on the banned list. "No, I can't eat that either," putting it back on the shelf with a sigh and turning toward the potato bread. It earns sympathy for your deprivation, admiration for your discipline, and indulgence for your complex personal needs. There's a way that melancholy is pleasurable and self-pity sweet. Combine that with self-righteousness, and you have a whole schedule of emotions to enjoy.

There's a kind of subtle pleasure in intentional deprivation. It might be worth doing just for the raw enjoyment of it—especially if you didn't pretend that it was virtuous. But today I feel as guilty about that pleasure as I once felt about indulging. One friend calls it "indulging in self-denial."

Puritanism also involves a kind of roller coaster of sin and redemption. The rules are so strict that most people will fall off the path from time to time. This leads to guilt, repentance, and ultimately a return to virtue. Therapist Ellen Montague describes how the same cycle occurs with food: "One reason I adopted an extreme diet in the first place is that in some ways I am most comfortable when I am feeling bad about myself. It's the most familiar way. It's harder and scarier to love myself.

"There is practically no better place to play this out than in the food arena. Every meal I almost always get a chance to feel bad about myself and the choices I make. Then I can make up for it by some act of severity on myself and feel good until the next 'mistake.' "

One test to see if puritanism is a hidden motive for you is to imagine what it would be like if healthy foods were precisely the ones you craved. Would it still be any fun? Or would you have to come up with a new diet, one that produced a satisfactory feeling of self-punishment and constant temptations to "cheat."

Creating an Identity

The essence of orthorexia is the way in which it makes food carry unnecessary burdens. Food as spirituality, food as self-denial, food as substitute for the chaotic world, food as guarantee against ever getting sick—in all these food is carrying a weight too heavy for its nature. Yes, food is important, but not that important. There is much more than food being squeezed onto your plate.

Besides all these large issues that fall on food, there is another important one to consider, the sense of identity. You can base your understanding of who you are on how you eat. Even so generic (and generally healthy) a food theory as vegetarianism can provide this: "Hi, I'm a vegetarian, pleased to meet you." It's even more so with more complex food theories. If you follow macrobiotics, you are a "macro," very likely all your friends are too, and you want the rest of the world to join as well. It is very relieving to be able to say, "I'm a macro." It's so much more comforting than to have to say, "I'm a person with lots of different needs and characteristics; I can't really pin down who I am." The latter is more honest, but the first has a delightfully shrink-wrapped character that leaves aside questing and confusion.

A food theory can expand to contain many more elements of identity than the bare fact of what you eat. Vegetarianism, for example, has a political aspect: the undeniably valid point that it is much more efficient to use land to grow human food than to grow animal feed and give it to animals raised for slaughter. It would become easy to produce enough food to feed everyone on earth far into the next century if everyone could be induced to become vegetarian.

Indeed, it's hard to fault a teenager or other young idealistic person who takes on a set of food beliefs as a way to find him- or herself; actually, I highly respect it, if only because the qualities of self-discipline and delayed gratification that food theories develop are wonderful to see in a person growing up in today's world. However, after a while it would be nice to develop a sense of self that doesn't depend primarily on what you eat.

The use of food to establish identity is certainly not peculiar only to orthorexia. Major world religions have included dietary rules for millennia. I grew up Jewish, a tradition famous for its restrictions regarding diet. Although the branch I belonged to, Reform Judaism, was not strict, I passed through a period of trying out such strictness to see what it felt like.

As most people know, traditional Judaism forbids certain foods, based on prohibitions in the Old Testament. Pork is off-limits, as are all types of shellfish, and it is illegal to combine milk and meat. Vegetarian food, interestingly, is automatically kosher, although one can keep kosher without being a vegetarian.

There are many arguments regarding why these rules should have been promulgated to the ancient Israelites. The one I prefer points out that most of the rules are basically sensible. Pork can carry diseases such as trichinosis, and shellfish can cause fatal allergic reactions, so avoiding them simply makes sense. However, the prohibition against mixing milk and meat is not so easy to explain from this perspective, and the ethical argument must be made that it is cruel to, as it prohibits in the Bible, "boil a kid in its mother's milk."

But looking back now, it seems clear to me that there are altogether different motivations behind eating kosher, and they obviously overlap with orthorexia. Dietary restrictions establish an identity.

For a religion to exist, its members have to have a way of distinguishing themselves from people who are not members. Otherwise it's only a philosophy, and you might be unclear on whether you belonged to a certain religion or not. It's a more serious issue than joining a club with a secret handshake.

Having dietary rules is a very effective way to establish boundaries. I can only imagine that their self-imposed limitations gave the Israelites a clear sense that they were definitely distinct from, and also highly superior to, their neighbors, who freely indulged in "unclean" foods. In any case, I felt that way when I briefly followed the rules of kosher eating as an adolescent. I was in harness; I was carrying a yoke on my shoulders, a yoke that made me feel important, special, and perhaps most of all, a Very Good Person for obeying the rules. What a relief from all the confusion of being a teenager! By fighting against my own impulses and obeying a difficult set of dietary restrictions, I had belonging, righteousness, self-discipline, and identity all sewn up.

Although my fascination with kosher eating lasted only a short time, the feeling came back when I turned to raw-foodism. Indeed, it was with a familiar feeling that I put on this new yoke, and the familiar comfort came with it. I was a raw-foodist, clearly superior to my neighbors who gorged themselves on cooked vegetables, a member of a group that would instantly accept me regardless of my character simply because I ate the way they did (I was an extremely annoying person at the time, so this was good).

I had no problems opening a conversation with raw-foodist women. "Let's go pick some wild sorrel," I would say, and straightaway I'd have a companion for a wander into the woods.

When I would feel temptations to eat a hot dog or a pizza, the act of suppressing that desire had a deep sweetness to it. I was making the "right" choice, one that my conscience and my peer group would approve. The more difficult it was to stick to, the more enjoyable would feel the act of renunciation.

However, there is a huge difference between a sense of identity based on food and a religious identity that includes food rules as distinguishing feature. Judaism, like other religions with dietary restrictions, is obviously far more than diet. Religious faith, history, tradition, culture, philosophy, and so much more go into a religion; in a food trip there's mostly just food. One expands the soul, the other flattens it.

Again there's an easy test to see if your orthorexia contains aspects of identity seeking. Imagine that everyone in the world ate the same way you do. Would you still want to do it?

Fear of Other People
While foods can serve to give you an identity in a group, they can also do just the opposite: keep you separated from any possible group. If you eat strangely enough, you pretty much have to eat by yourself. This can provide a wonderful excuse for isolation if underneath it all you are afraid of other people anyway.

The one food theory that most commonly leads to social isolation is that of food allergies. No one is going to share your personal food allergies, so you can easily belong to a group of one. Besides, food allergies themselves represent a kind of fear of the outside world. Your body has become intolerant of many innocent foods; this, in a sense, symbolizes a general intolerance for life. The more you delve into food allergies, the more you restrict what you eat, the more your body becomes a prima donna. You begin to turn down everything and everyone; you'd rather stay at home with your spelt bread and rice bran sweetener than face the harsh world with its superabundant and intolerable wheat.

The process of using food as a means of isolation may not be conscious. You may simply feel that you are following a healthy diet; it may seem that you regret the isolation that it imposes on you. However, beneath the surface you may be acting out a different drama.

Test yourself: Imagine that you suddenly knew hundreds of people who eat just like you. Would you be happy to share your meals with them? Or are you secretly pleased by having an excuse to keep to yourself?

Of course, there's nothing wrong with wanting to spend time alone. But if you are using food as an excuse to cut off contact with others, at the very least you are playing a dishonest game with yourself. In general it's much healthier to face what's going on honestly.

WHAT DO ALL THESE HIDDEN AGENDAS HAVE IN COMMON?

While each is unique, taken together all the motivations described in this chapter share some common tendencies. They all involve using food as more than food, laying a weight on diet that diet shouldn't have to carry, using food as a symbol for identity, spirituality, and safety. This extra weight riding on food pulls the energy and emotion out of other, more important parts of your life.

In fact, it is transferring too much of life's meaning onto food that makes orthorexia an eating disorder. If you simply eat healthy food but don't give it more of a place in your life than it's really due, you have a good diet—a laudable goal. But when you use food to drain away the energy from other parts of your life, you are impoverishing your soul. Instead of dealing with your real feelings—your real challenges, interests, desires and needs—you pretend to find them in food. You transfer anxiety over how your life is going to anxiety over what you are going to eat. It certainly seems a lot less threatening. But it's an escape and a way of fooling yourself.

WHAT TO DO?

Do you recognize yourself in any of the above discussion? Do you see any traits of orthorexia in your approach to food? If you do, you may wonder whether you can do anything to escape from the trap of health food obsession. And then your mind will probably answer back, "But it's so good for me. It's what I have to do." The underlying nervousness you feel, the sense of conviction that maybe you are doing some things wrong, gets buried beneath the propaganda of your favorite diet.

To help you take the next step, I'd like to first counter some of that propaganda, to show how the sacred principles of your favorite dietary approach are more arbitrary, less perfect, less nobly true than they might seem. It is not my intention to indicate that diet doesn't matter at all—far from it. I'd just like to weaken its hold a little, to show you that all the advice you have read is less certain, less absolute, less impeccable than you think. It still may be good for you, but it's not profound enough to claim your full attention.

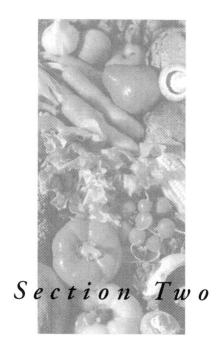

Section Two

The
HEALING
DIETS

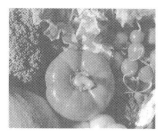

It was 1975. I was living alone for the first time, and this was my first real dinner party. Although I felt a bit exposed and scared, everyone seemed to like my sparsely decorated house, with its surrealist posters, Indian-print fabrics, and red wax candles. I was just beginning to feel that I had made a success of stepping into the post-hippie world when suddenly I heard a scream from the kitchen.

I ran in to see what was wrong. Beverly, a tall massage therapist with hair to her waist, stood looking into my cupboards.

"Look what's in here!" she cried to the gathering crowd.

I peered forward, expecting to find a tarantula, or at least a dead rat. But all I saw was the usual stuff. Rows of canned food.

"See what he's got in his cupboards!" she announced to ten people looking over her shoulders. To my astonishment, I heard gasps of disgust.

"Steven," one of my guests said accusingly, "you don't really eat this garbage, do you?"

I gave her a blank look. I knew I must be doing something horribly wrong, but I didn't know what.

Beverly picked up one of the cans and hefted it sorrowfully. "Beef stew. Nalley's Beef Stew, no less. Don't you know what this stuff does to you?"

I suddenly understood. I had purchased the wrong food!

Apparently this was a part of the rules of my new world that I hadn't recognized. I still didn't know the specifics, but the general principle was clear: Everything I thought I knew about food was wrong.

"I don't really know much about food," I said. "But I want to." Beverly smiled. By the end of the evening all my cans stood in a pile at the door of the Salvation Army while my cupboards were filled with jars full of unrecognizable (but quite pretty) beans, grains, seaweeds, and dried fruits.

That evening began my initiation into the world of healthy eating. I was a quick learner. Within a year I had surpassed my teachers and become an organic farmer and a raw foods enthusiast. I believed that all foods should be eaten in their raw and natural state. To Beverly and her friends this was cool beyond belief, and I basked in their approval.

But after about six months, as I sat in the middle of a field of carrots chewing my plateful of raw veggies, I heard a grunt from behind me. It was Mr. Lux, a well-known lecturer on macrobiotics. He had arrived that afternoon, preparatory to his lecture the following morning.

"Don't you know what that stuff does to you?" he asked.

"Makes me incredibly healthy?" I replied.

"Absolutely not!" he shouted. "Raw vegetables are too yin. They cause arthritis and cancer."

That was a shock. But I recognized his superior knowledge, just as I had intuitively surrendered to Beverly's. Here was a wisdom about eating that trumped everything I'd ever known. It was the wisdom of Japan, Eastern food theory, far advanced beyond the crude food beliefs of the West. Within a month I ate only brown rice and cooked vegetables, to the great admiration of my new friends on the farm.

My macrobiotic regimen went on unchecked for almost a year. I spent hours slicing vegetables prior to lightly sautéing them; I purchased Japanese delicacies such as umeboshi plums and seitan, and I generally prided myself on my discerning ability to recognize the truth against the background noise of untrue beliefs.

Then a famous acupuncturist and master of Chinese medicine came through town. Master Le Quiong belonged to a family that for twelve generations had practiced the healing arts of China. Even Mao, it was said, consulted his wisdom in time of need. Feeling greatly honored to have the opportunity, I made an appointment to ask his advice on a few mild health problems that had developed since I'd started to eat healthy foods.

Master Le Quiong asked me to describe my diet. When I'd finished, he smiled, no doubt in approval. I was used to receiving such approval, because I was by far the most religious eater on the farm, and I further assumed that because it was also from the East, Chinese dietary theory should follow macrobiotics closely. I awaited his benediction.

"Very bad diet," he said.

At first I didn't hear.

"Very bad way to eat. My opinion, you eat like a crazy man," he continued. "Will get bad sick. My opinion, you need eat meat. I recommend you eat beef. Beef stew. You ever heard of Nalley's Beef Stew? Very good for you."

The world swam before my eyes. My certainty vanished; I no longer knew what was true about diet, nor whose opinion I should please. It was the first time I had closed the circle and found that dietary theories contradict, the first time I realized it was more complicated than The One Right Way to Eat and The One Wrong Way to Eat.

I wasn't yet cured. I would still adopt several other dietary theories before I gave up entirely five years later, but it was the beginning of the end.

THE UNIVERSAL COOKBOOK

I used to fantasize about writing a universal cookbook for eating theorists. Each food would come complete with a citation from one system or authority claiming it the most divine edible ever created and another, from an opposing view, damning it as the worst pestilence one human being ever fed to another.

This would be very easy. For example, a famous concept derived from the Western naturopathic tradition proclaims that raw fruits and vegetables are the ideal foods. Some proponents of this school exclaim periodically, "The greatest enemy of man is the cooking stove!" In contrast, Eastern food theories in general ban raw foods as unhealthy, attributing to their consumption such illnesses as MS, rheumatoid arthritis, and cancer.

Similar discrepancies abound in alternative dietary medicine. The following rules may be found in one or another food theory:

Whole grains are the staff of life (traditional naturopathy). Grains increase insulin secretion (Zone diet).

Spicy food is bad (traditional naturopathy, Asian medical theory). Cayenne peppers are health-promoting (some forms of traditional naturopathy).

Fasting on oranges is healthy (raw-foodism). Citrus fruits are too acidic (some forms of traditional naturopathy).

Fruits are the ideal food (traditional naturopathy, raw foodism, fruitarianism). Fruit causes candida (candida theory).

Milk is good only for young cows, and pasteurized milk is even worse (traditional naturopathy). Boiled milk "is the food of the gods" (traditional Hindu health belief).

Foods should be eaten in their whole, unrefined state, and refined foods are bad for you (traditional naturopathy). Everyone needs to take vitamin pills—which are, actually, the most highly refined foods you can imagine (modern naturopathy).

Fermented foods, such as sauerkraut and vinegar, are essentially rotten (traditional Hindu health belief). Fermented foods aid digestion (macrobiotics, some branches of traditional naturopathy), and apple cider vinegar is the cure for all diseases (some branches of traditional naturopathy).

Sweets are bad (naturopathy, Chinese medicine, dental theory). Honey is nature's most perfect food (some branches of traditional naturopathy).

Butter is bad (modern medicine, naturopathy). Clarified butter is health-promoting (some aspects of Ayurvedic medicine).

Proteins should not be combined with starches (food-combining theory). Adzuki beans and brown rice should always be cooked together (macrobiotics).

When I first began to discover these contradictions I found ways to explain them away. The most obvious was that one dietary theory was right and all the others were wrong.

IS THERE A RIGHT WAY TO EAT?

Of course diet matters. By showing all these contradictions, it is not my intention to suggest that diet does not matter at all, that all dietary choices are equally arbitrary and insane. There is no question, for example, that the standard American diet is unhealthy and that well-balanced vegetarianism is much better for you. What is insane, however, is the fanaticism and certainty that attaches to dietary theories. Let's face it, everyone is different, and what works well for one person may not work so well for another. (The Eat Right for Your Type diet attempts to capitalize in a simplistic way on this very fact. See Chapter 11.)

Unfortunately, the reality is that it's hard to find out for sure. Maybe you feel best in the short term on diet A but might live longer on diet B. No food theorist really knows; there is a whole lot of hot air blowing through the grave dietary pronouncements of macrobiotics, raw foods theory, and every other approach to diet.

It's impossible to know for sure what one should eat. But rather than admit that the situation is murky, each food theory tends to posture as the One True Food Religion, the sacred and secret source of life-giving dietary rules. It's a seductive concept but one that is made somewhat hard to take too seriously when you realize that another theory has staked opposing claims with equal gravity. When you see how wildly the theories differ, it all begins to look a little arbitrary—just as when each side of a battle prays to God for victory and somehow assumes that the other side has no right to a similar prayer.

Maybe one of these eating theories has a monopoly on truth and all the others are wrong, but I would suggest that actually it goes the other way: None of them has a monopoly on truth. Each is just a piece of the truth, worthy of consideration but not veneration.

In the next nine chapters, I will briefly introduce the main dietary theories, discuss what it is about them that can so capture the imagination, and suggest a less fanatical attitude toward their insights.

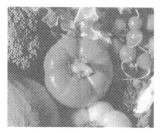

6.

Food Allergies
and Imperfection

Food allergy treatment can be a powerful healing approach that at times appears to reduce symptoms dramatically in practically any illness. By identifying what foods you are allergic to and eliminating them from your diet, you stand a chance of improving such diseases as asthma, rheumatoid arthritis, migraine headaches, Crohn's disease—indeed, almost any disease you can think of. Unfortunately, this broadly effective treatment can also turn out to be a royal road to orthorexia.

There are two kinds of food allergies: the immediate-onset type, which can lead to hives and potentially fatal swelling of the lips, face, tongue, and throat; and a much more gradual form that causes relatively subtle symptoms. Shrimp allergy is an example of the former. Children with this allergy have died simply from walking into a house where shrimp are cooking. As with a bee sting allergy, the only remedy for this type of dramatic allergic response is a timely injection of adrenaline. Peanuts and strawberries are other common triggers for allergies of this type.

The other form of food allergy does not show itself so rapidly. Rather, over a period of weeks or months, constant exposure to a food allergen may cause fatigue, runny nose, headache, or any of numerous other relatively mild symptoms. Because allergies of this type are vague, subjective, and hard to document, conventional medicine has tended to ignore them entirely. It's not so much that physicians don't believe that these delayed-type food allergies exist; rather, they find them too indistinct to grapple with and would therefore prefer not to think about them at all. For this reason food allergies have fallen into the realm of alternative medicine, which is not deterred by vagueness or subjectivity.

There is very little doubt in my mind that identifying and eliminating a few primary allergens can sometimes significantly improve health. The trick is finding out just what foods you need to reject, since effects that take place over weeks are rather hard to pin down.

The ultimate food allergen identification method starts by eliminating all foods but turkey and white rice (two foods that are famously nonallergenic). After a month or so of this epicurean delight, you add in one new food and stick to this three-item menu for another couple of weeks. If there are no adverse effects, you add another, and so on, until you find what you can and cannot eat successfully.

However, few people have the cast-iron will to follow such a program. Therefore, numerous methods have been invented that purport to identify allergenic foods. Some of the more popular include blood tests with various acronyms such as RAST or ALCAT. Another famous method involves a special machine that measures the electrical resistance of your skin, sends it to a computer, and spits out pages of detailed information. Then there's applied kinesiology, in which you hold a vial of a certain food in one hand and a practitioner tests your strength in the other. Most of these methods have not passed impartial validation tests, which require at the very least that if the same test is done twice on the same person, the results will come out the same. None seems to work particularly well in real life, and many are notoriously unreliable.

Nonetheless, because it is so arduous to follow the elimination approach, these tests are very popular, and they yield reams of highly specific suggestions on what you should and should not eat. Usually these are ranked by severity of response. Foods that rank high are supposed to require permanent elimination from the diet, while those of lesser allergenicity can still be consumed, but on a rotating basis. In my experience these test results seem to range from moderately accurate to entirely off base.

Certain foods are more frequently allergenic than others. Milk is the most common allergen, and it is well known to many pediatricians that a substantial percentage of children with asthma, frequent colds, or eczema will improve if dairy products are taken out of the diet. (If you try this, don't forget to supply your child with sufficient calcium from another source.) Canker sores often respond to the elimination of wheat, and stomach pain to the removal of milk or soy.

If you can achieve good results through the elimination of just a few foods, the food allergy approach can only be seen as wonderful. But too often we can't stop there. We need (or believe we need) to eliminate dozens of foods to achieve the improvement we desire. Worse still, over time the list usually grows rather than shrinks, and eventually almost everything edible falls off. We come to view the world of edibles as a minefield of dangerous enemies rather than a collection of good-tasting treats.

Too often food allergies come to monopolize all the mental space of those who focus on them. Not content to improve a few specific symptoms, the food allergy follower begins to place blame for every ache and pain and even every annoying emotion on the head of food allergies. There's no stopping the progression. Last month it was chocolate and headaches (a reasonable association). Now if my big toe twinges for a second, it's due to that avocado I ate yesterday. Have I developed a cavity? Blame it on lentils. I even knew a man who blamed his divorce on food allergies. The way he tells it, he ate an off-limits raisin, which caused a flare-up of allergenic cravings that made him binge on bread, in consequence of which his brain chemistry became altered and he yelled at his wife. The next thing he knew, they were divorced. (She tells the story a bit differently.)

After a while food allergies come to run your life completely. For Patty it took more than a year to progress from voluntarily using these techniques to improve her health to the point where she was enslaved by them. Her story began in 1992. It was an unhealthy time for Patty. She caught colds eight or nine times that year, and with each one she stayed sick for a week or more.

Each time she got sick, Patty ended up on one or another antibiotic, most of which would trigger galloping yeast infections. It was really getting her down. Her conventional doctor wasn't much help, because conventional medicine doesn't have any proven techniques to break the cycle of frequent colds.

Increasingly desperate, Patty began to scour the pages of magazines devoted to vitamins, herbs, and other unconventional approaches to healing. She tried a few recommendations, such as zinc and vitamin C, but without any notable effect. One day an article about food allergies caught her attention. It read as if it were talking to her personally.

"Do you get sinus infections, excessive mucus, fatigue, or stomachaches? If so, you need to get checked for food allergies." The page showed a woman with dark circles under her eyes and an itchy red nose.

"You can restore your health without taking drugs," it went on. "Learn about this side-effect-free, natural approach to taking charge of your life."

Patty went right out and bought a book on food allergies. The more she read, the more excited she became. Even before she finished the book, Patty quit drinking milk. The effects were dramatic. It took about a month for her to see the difference, but by that time her head felt clearer, and she wasn't blowing her nose all the time. When February came and went without a cold, she knew she was onto something.

Patty stayed healthy through March as well—a record-two month stretch without a cold. But when it began to rain in April, she felt the familiar rasp in her throat and the leaden tiredness behind her eyes. It was a cold coming on, and instead of feeling grateful that she had stayed well longer than usual, Patty fell back into a sea of despair. But only briefly. She soon decided that she simply hadn't eliminated enough foods and that now she needed to cut out wheat.

Dairy-free and wheatless, Patty stayed healthy for three months, but in July she came down sick again. This time she decided to seek professional help. A little research identified a local "holistic" doctor who claimed to specialize in food allergies. She underwent the testing he recommended and soon received a sheet of paper listing six major allergies, nineteen minor allergies, and seventy-two possible allergies.

Patty eliminated only the foods on the "major allergy" list: besides milk and wheat, also eggs, cheese, soy, corn, oats, and bananas. Whenever she purchased anything, she needed to read the label closely to see if it contained even a drop of the forbidden foods. She soon learned how to cook in accordance with the new rules.

This diet did set up enormous limitations on her life. Eating out at restaurants was impossible, and when she visited a friend she always had to bring her own food. However, she felt great and didn't catch cold again till September.

Patty knew what she had to do next. She pulled the list out of her file cabinet and read the nineteen minor allergies. By the next day she had eliminated avocados, broccoli, tuna, safflower oil, apples, cabbage, butter, spinach, oregano, tomatoes, and nine other foods. She felt better already.

It was extremely hard to prepare a coherent meal now, and she had to spend hours every day figuring out how to balance her nutrition while still sticking to her diet. Nonetheless, she faithfully adhered to the regimen. It seemed that her life depended on it.

Certainly her body depended on it. After a few months she found that if she accidentally consumed even one of her most minor allergens she would develop a significant reaction, ranging from headaches to debilitating fatigue. That had never happened before. It was as if her body, freed from enduring allergenic foods, had lost all its ability to tolerate them. She had to eat perfectly. Oh, sometimes she "cheated," eating a slice of bread or half a can of tuna. But she paid for each indiscretion, or so she thought, with days of discomfort. Also, each time she would feel soiled, as if she had sinned, and would take a vow never to stray again.

Patty was so pleased with the changes in her life that she made her eight-year-old daughter get tested for allergies, too. She found seven major allergens and twelve minor ones, and Patty took them all away. Her ex-husband protested, but Patty got Amanda on her side by talking up all the advantages of the new way of eating. "You don't want your insides all gummed up, do you?" she said, and Amanda's eyes grew wide.

It didn't stop there. Whenever a friend got sick, Patty would deliver the lecture. "Admit it," she would say. "You're allergic to something. You've got to stop sticking anything in your mouth that catches your fancy. You've got to be more careful." Not that she had many friends left. She would catch people eating whatever was put in front of them and shake her head as if she'd caught them on a drunken binge.

She still caught about three colds a year. Nonetheless, that was a lot better than when she had started. Patty knew that what she was doing was right, and her "holistic" doctor thought so, too. "You're one of my best patients," he said.

Patty was satisfied. Her doctor was more than satisfied. However, was this a side-effect-free treatment as the book had promised? Patty was certainly healthier, at least so far as colds went. But was she really healthier overall? Was her life better?

Consider the cost that the identification and avoidance of food allergens had entailed. Patty had no friends. Her daughter was forced to choose each food she ate off a list and could never share ice cream, cake, peanut butter, or chocolate with a friend. Patty's whole day was spent arranging dietary matters. She couldn't even look at an apple, an orange, or a zucchini without feeling ill. Is this wellness? Isn't obsession a side effect? Shouldn't her holistic doctor have been interested enough in Patty as a whole person to keep this in mind?

To me it seemed as if Patty's life had been destroyed. If only she had stopped with the dairy or the dairy and wheat. When she eliminated those, she felt better, even if not perfectly better. In her continued quest to eliminate every single symptom, she had made herself a thoroughgoing orthorexic, and at least a little crazy.

HOW TO USE FOOD ALLERGY TREATMENT SUCCESSFULLY

In my medical practice I must have seen at least fifty people like Patty, and many more who were at least halfway as obsessed. I eventually came to regard food allergy treatment as the equivalent of a dangerous medication, one that should be prescribed only sparingly. I began counseling my patients who were interested in food allergies to use the treatment in moderation to keep down the "side effects." It's like taking the lowest possible dose of a medication known to cause drowsiness. "Don't try to get perfectly healthy" became my standard line. "Just cut out at most three or four foods and appreciate the benefits that come from doing that much." Trying to get everything perfect by eliminating more foods always seems to backfire. Not only does the body become progressively more of a prima donna, but your life will take on so many strange alterations that it becomes increasingly questionable which is worse, the cure or the disease.

A BAND-AID SOLUTION

Is wheat actually an evil food? Is corn? Is soy? These three common food allergens are not toxic like alcohol, nor necessarily polluted with food preservatives and artificial colors. Soy is even popularly described in other healing systems as a miracle healing food. Yet they are at the top of the allergenic list. To be fair about it, if you are allergic to these innocent foods, the problem is in you, not in the food.

In other words, removing food allergens from the diet is a Band-Aid treatment. It doesn't get to the root of the problem, the root being "Why can't my body handle these perfectly good foods?" This is ironic, because practitioners of holistic medicine love to accuse conventional medicine of treating the symptom and ignoring the cause of the illness. One of the key alternative medicine phrases goes, "If you just treat the symptoms and ignore the cause, the cause will keep right on chewing away at you, and soon you will have new symptoms."

But isn't this precisely what happens with food allergies? When you treat the symptom by removing an otherwise innocent food that your body can't tolerate, the internal process of intolerance goes on unabated, and soon you are allergic to numerous other foods. If you cut out wheat and corn and eggs, soon you will be allergic to oats and barley and raisins.

Not that I have an alternative. There doesn't seem to be any good way to get to the root of food allergies and heal them from within. Although food allergen identification and avoidance is a superficial treatment, it is often the only solution available. However, you need to keep in mind that this is nothing like a perfect treatment. It is a symptomatic treatment with a host of fairly severe side effects.

Still, cutting out the most allergenic foods from your diet is often a very sensible, practical step. It won't cure you, but it may make you feel better, like staying indoors while the cottonwoods bloom. Trying to avoid everything allergenic forever, though, is like going to live in a cave to overcome hay fever; it may work, but the cost is a bit high.

ACCEPTING IMPERFECTION

Psychologically, food allergies involve a kind of intolerance of all discomfort, all imperfection in the body. I don't know which comes first, the allergies or the intolerance, but the net effect is a personality that holds little tolerance for any mood, discomfort, or disturbance. In a sense we become picky eaters at every level, not only of food but of all sensations.

Do you really need to have a body that is absolutely, perfectly healthy and a mind that is never troubled or upset? Do you really prefer spending the rest of your life warding off dangerously tempting foods over catching the occasional cold? Do you really get as sick from minor allergens as you allow yourself to believe? How much of it do you exaggerate, even to yourself? Does it warm your heart to shake your head sadly and say, "No, I can't eat that. It makes the skin on my third toe turn red." Could some of it be psychosomatic, a mental effect caused by your strong opinions against certain foods?

It took years for Patty to admit to herself that she wasn't quite so allergic as she made out. Yes, milk, wheat, and—as it turned out—peanuts, definitely made her ill. But she eventually concluded that she'd puffed up her reactions to other foods in order to feel vulnerable and fragile.

It also took years for Patty to find other ways to give herself love besides pretending she felt more miserable than she did, other ways to acknowledge her vulnerabilities and take care of her needs. As she learned this, she gradually caught the knack of tolerating an imperfect body. It wasn't that she stopped having allergic reactions. Rather, she found that by taking better care of her feelings, she could easily tolerate minor aches and pains. Today she eats most everything except milk, wheat, and peanuts, and although she occasionally feels tired or has a mild headache, she doesn't think about it. As for colds, she gets about two a year, and they are mild.

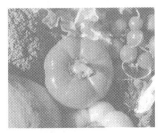

7.

Back to Eden with Raw Foods Theory

After food allergies, perhaps the next most common alternative path to orthorexia is raw foods theory. Its origin reaches back to the early 1800s, but this extreme dietary theory continues to attract converts today. From Jeremy Safron's incredibly successful Raw Experience restaurant in San Francisco to the neoreligious incantations of *Nature's First Law*, raw-foodism offers a consistent and strangely compelling vision of dietary redemption. Raw foods theory was my personal entry into orthorexia twenty-five years ago, and I retain a certain fondness for its wild assertions.

As the name implies, this enduring theory of eating revolves around consuming foods raw: raw fruits, raw vegetables, and even raw grains. The story of raw-foodism begins at the spas and sanitariums of early-nineteenth-century Europe, when a reaction against the industrial transformations of life led to what was perhaps the first stirrings of the "back to nature" movement. Jean-Jacques Rousseau had started it a few decades before, with his idealization of the Natural State. This impulse was taken up with particular enthusiasm in Germany, by such people as Father Sebastian Kneipp, whose "nature cure" involved outdoor life, simple diet, fasting, and "baths" in the sun, wind, water, and earth. In America, Sylvester Graham (of Graham cracker fame), John Harvey Kellogg (of Kellogg cereal fame), and later Jethro Kloss and Gaylord Hauser spread a similar message.

The point was simple and well taken. In those days factories were just beginning to replace farms, canned food to substitute for fresh vegetables, sedentary existence in dim buildings to push out healthy outdoor exercise. The world was losing its way in a forest of smokestacks, and over the decades leading up to the present, this trend has only continued. The great turning-away of civilization from nature called up ranks of prophets, prophets of nature who wished to instill repentance and restore the right way of life. This natural health movement they created is the direct antecedent not only of contemporary alternative medicine but also of organic farming, natural foods in general, and even environmentalism.

Natural health philosophies went by many names, but nearly all enlisted the word "nature" in their titles. Examples include Natural Medicine, Nature's Laws of Healing, the Nature Cure and Natural Hygiene. At the turn of the century, a German immigrant and disciple of Father Kneipp named Benedict Lust coined another term that persists up to today: naturopathy. Lust also founded the world's first health food store, in New York City.

We owe to naturopathic fervor many of the preventive health concepts that we now take for granted. Naturopathic physicians promoted the then-radical notion that disease could be prevented by eating a diet low in fat and rich in whole grains and fresh fruits and vegetables, combined with healthy lifestyle and avoidance of chemical toxins. Today this is the standard doctrine of conventional medicine, too, but for many decades it ran counter to trends and was systematically denounced by medical authorities.

Modern naturopathic physicians (NDs) seldom focus on raw foods anymore. Herbs and food supplements are now more the staple of naturopathic treatment, probably because, as pills, they are more agreeable to modern people. But natural healing began with a focus on raw foods, and this school of eating embodies many of the deepest instincts of natural medicine.

Clearly, before it is cooked, a carrot is more in its natural state than afterward. A simple test proves it: You can plant a raw carrot and it will grow, while a cooked carrot will not. Intuitively, therefore, a raw carrot has more "life energy" in it than a cooked one. Even a cooked carrot has more life energy than a canned carrot that has been embalmed for two or three years. Some foods, such as vinegar and meat, are felt to go the other way and provide more death energy than life energy. A modern offshoot of raw foods theory, sometimes called "instincto," seeks its quantum of life energy in raw meat; I don't know if any school yet follows the dictum expressed in a Broadway version of the Dracula story that I once saw, in which live flies and mice are extolled for the same reason as raw carrots.

The essence of raw-foodism is an intuitive, spiritual concept and one that is shared by many cultures. In Chinese medicine day-old food is considered "wrecked"; it has no *qi* (a Chinese term somewhat similar to "life force"). In the dietary and medical beliefs of India, foods either have or do not have *prana,* another loose synonym for "life force," and raw fruits, vegetables and nuts have the most.

But over the last century, scientific arguments have become more influential than semispiritual ones. For this reason proponents of raw foods have often tried to bolster their faith in rawness by claiming that raw foods surpass other food choices because of the many enzymes they contain. These enzymes are said to offer numerous health benefits, from improving digestion to fighting all the diseases of old age.

Actually, this notion is just a leftover from the nineteenth-century understanding of biochemistry. It is true that there are many enzymes in raw foods, but since they are curdled by the acid found in the stomach anyway, it's hard to see how they could really make any difference. But under the belief that a scientific-sounding expression is necessary to build credibility, this enzyme canard never gets left out of raw foods literature. However, it's just a distraction. The raw foods diet is not really a hankering after enzymes. It is a spiritual quest, translated from the invisible arena of the heart and soul into the more obvious and visible frontier of the body.

BACK TO THE NATURAL STATE

Whether stated or not, the raw foods diet embodies a nostalgic longing to return to the Natural State, assumed to have existed in preindustrial civilization. Jethro Kloss, in his classic *Back to Eden* (Public Domain Edition, Woodbridge Press, 1981), makes this underlying orientation clear. Originally published in the 1930s, this book played a central role in the natural health revival of the 1960s, and it wonderfully captures the authentic tone of early natural medicine proponents. Kloss's language is more Christian than might be in vogue today among raw food theorists, but the essence of what he says remains at the root of all raw food thinking.

For Kloss the quest for natural living is clearly nothing less than the desire to rediscover the innocence of the beginning. "Since Eve first surrendered to appetite," he writes, "man has been growing more and more self-indulgent, until health is being sacrificed on the altar of appetite." The prophetic tone Kloss uses here suggests a need for repentance, for atonement, for returning to the ways of righteousness. As we will see below, the popular modern work *Nature's First Law* continues to strike the prophetic bell.

Kloss frequently tells us that our health depends on living in harmony with nature's laws and receiving the gifts implanted in the world by an all-wise deity who fills the soil with every substance necessary for building of our bodies. (Today natural health writers would say that soils have become depleted due to artificial fertilizers, but this hadn't yet been recognized in Kloss's day.)

Kloss goes on to tell us that bad eating habits and the use of refined and adulterated foods are largely responsible for not only all the sickness but the social ills of the world as well.

Some of Kloss's statements have become accepted wisdom today. For example: "Although food may be ample in quantity, modern methods of refining remove the most important elements, and in many cases they are adulterated, and preservatives added to conceal their inferior quality." This statement was radical when Kloss enunciated it, but you wouldn't find much disagreement nowadays.

He puts it more strongly elsewhere: "the refined, degerminated, demineralized and devitalized foods are a curse to humanity." Here again we return to the food equivalent of original sin and the need for repentance, so that we can go back to Eden.

Much of Kloss's tone can be seen in contemporary works on raw foods. For example, as Ann Wigmore writes in *The Hippocrates Diet and Health Program* (Avery Publishing, 1984):

"There is much historical evidence to show that mankind first evolved in a climate that supported his every need. Without weapons for killing and fire for cooking, man lived mainly on the fruits, leaves shoots, roots, seeds, and nuts that were abundant. . . . Only thousands of years later did man begin to move north, and having discovered fire, cook his food. Since then, and for thousands of years, we have cooked food, and . . . our health has continued to decline as a result."

In the second half of this passage, the explicit attack on cooked food begins. This principle, which can already be seen implicitly in Kloss, becomes a violent enthusiasm among modern raw food advocates. Consider *Nature's First Law*, a recent manifesto of raw foodism by raw foods religionists Stephen Arlin, Fouad Dini, and David Wolfe (Maul Brothers Publishing, 1998). It features the three authors, naked on the cover, concealed by the leaves of a tree, eating fruit. Its grand language vilifies the practice of cooking food with a passion that seems ludicrous to someone who doesn't share the same assumptions.

"It is very difficult to explain something of this majesty and glory to closed and indoctrinated minds," begins this scripture of the religion of raw-foodism.

"So long as human beings persist in consuming cooked food, there can be neither real civilization nor lasting health on Earth." A strong claim, but it is only the beginning.

"Cooked food is the first and worst addiction. It is the physiochemical basis for all other addictions."

"The gravest terrorism is the terrorism inflicted upon children when they are forced to copy the cooked-food addictions of their parents."

And, repeated at the end of each of forty chapters, "Cooked food is poison."

Having not met the authors, I'm not sure how much of this is deliberate irony, but judging by the discussion on many Web sites, followers don't take it that way. Indeed, the religion of raw foods suggests that betrayal might be punishable by death (dealt out by God, not by the mild-mannered followers themselves); it has been widely noted in these discussion groups that T. C. Fry, one of the greatest evangelizers of raw foods, was punished by the raw foods gods when he turned to other foods. Ignoring the warnings of his friends, he fell sick and promptly died.

THE ENEMY: MEAT

Besides cooked food, the other great enemy is meat. As Jethro Kloss says, "Meats of all kinds are unnatural." Philosophically, the notion that meat is "unnatural" is a bit strange. Do coyotes, then, engage in an unnatural pursuit when they hunt down rabbits? Chimpanzees eat meat, and we are extraordinarily closely related to them. Unkind, yes, to those that are eaten, but hardly unnatural.

"Fish, fowl, and seafoods are very likely to contain numbers of germs. The bacteria infect the intestines, causing colitis and many other diseases. They always cause putrefaction." I will return to the notion of intestinal putrefaction below, when I discuss colonics. It is not so much a literal concept (the intestines are always filled to the brim with bacteria anyway) but a general sense of rotting from within, a vivid image of the evil that derives from eating the raw foods. It's Kloss as Cotton Mather, intestinal sinners in the hands of an angry God.

OVERCOMING SIN BY
CLEANSING THE BODY

In raw-foodism the religious longings to repent, to purify oneself, to return to a state of innocence are all transferred to diet. Going back to Eden means undoing the sins of civilization. "You have gone astray by eating putrefying meat and devitalized white flour," thunder the raw foods prophets. "Repent of your evil. Go, eat raw foods, and sin no more."

The sense of having gone astray and needing to return to the path of truth is universal to religions. Because raw-foodism is like a religion translated into physical terms, a spirituality expressed in terms of the body rather than the soul, this cleansing is a bit more . . . well, graphic than what would ordinarily be required in most other religions.

Rather than cleansing the soul with prayer, the raw-foodist may cleanse the body through enemas. The concept of colon cleansing has been closely allied with raw-foodism from the beginning. Back in the 1800s, enthusiasts such as John Harvey Kellogg (who thought that constipation, rather than the cooking stove, was the greatest enemy of health) tried hard to turn the nation's attention to its colons. Anticipating Freud but drawing physical rather than psychological consequences from toilet training, Kellogg insisted that "resisting the call of nature" was the cause of all degenerative diseases.

According to the theory of colon health that Kellogg helped develop, a lifetime of bad eating causes the colon to be caked with thick black lumps and a gray, concretelike material. This inner sludge is said to cause "autointoxication" as the colonic poisons seep through the colon wall into the body. This toxicity is the physical equivalent of evil; it must be flushed, washed, and scrubbed away before you can achieve the Kingdom of Good Health. Taking a few laxatives will not work. It is said to be gravely difficult to rid the body of this toxic sludge. Years of good diet might do it, but the most direct practice is the high enema, or colonic, the greatest of all inner purifications, capable of making your guts as fresh as those of Adam and Eve.

Colonics involve using a machine to pump water as high up in your colon as possible. For your edification and sense of accomplishment, the tubes used are transparent, so you can watch the residue flow out. All kinds of ugly-looking material passes by, presumed to be the toxic sludge of decades, the concrete caking your colon at last breaking free.

However, while there is probably nothing wrong with enemas, there is something quite wrong with the caked-colon theory. It's a rather fundamental error, although no one in the colon-health movement seems to have noticed. In a nutshell, there is nothing caking the lining of the colon.

Over the last decades conventional physicians have millions of times performed the procedure known as colonoscopy. This technique involves looking at the colon wall with a flexible telescope, in search of colon cancer. Keep in mind that among the patients usually examined by conventional physicians it is quite unlikely that very many have followed a raw foods or even vegetarian diet. Practically none have engaged in regular enemas. These colons under the telescope, therefore, should be thoroughly coated with a putrefying slime.

However, they're not coated with anything. I've watched colonoscopies. Nothing but clean pink flesh shows up through the scope. There's no sludge, no concrete, absolutely no accumulation at all.

This fact, one might think, would make the caked-colon concept somewhat hard to sustain. Nonetheless it persists. Every few years a new bestselling book makes the same untrue claim.

This is not to say that enemas couldn't have some value. Maybe they do. Perhaps enormous health benefits accrue, ones that simply have never been documented scientifically. But if they work, colonics do not do so by eliminating colonic sludge.

Colonics certainly do make one feel cleaned out. In fact, this may be the real driving force behind the theory of colon health: It feels good to get cleaned out from the inside. Actually, traditional natural medicine encourages us to clean everything else out, too— liver flushes, gallbladder flushes, kidney flushes, scrubbing the skin to remove toxins in the pores, and taking saunas and hot tubs to produce a cleansing sweat are all part of the same general principle. Lightness and emptiness are the physical sensations that characterize raw-foodism.

THE FEELING OF LIGHTNESS

In *The Unbearable Lightness of Being*, Milan Kundera wrote of the impulse to feel involved with life, to be bound to it by duty, necessity, and concern. Raw-foodists do not share this impulse. Whether consciously or unconsciously, they wish to float free from the weightiness of life on earth; they want to feel the body like an angel's body—weightless, transparent, saturated with light. Any hint of boundedness to physical reality is the enemy, whether it's a full stomach or a sensation of fatigue. The underlying script is "I don't really have a body at all. I'm pure spirit."

In this impulse orthorexia and anorexia overlap. In anorexia actual weight is the issue, while in raw-foodism it is the sensation of lightness, the physical feeling of not being weighed down to the earth that matter most. But the physical pleasure is the same, which can be quite intense (in a disembodied sort of way), and as Ellen Montague mentioned in Chapter 5, there may be more of a desire to lose weight in orthorexia than most orthorexics would like to admit.

Fasting is the ultimate route to feeling light. When you stop eating, you feel hungry for a couple of days, but then a different state takes over. You start to experience a sense of clearheadedness and increased mental and imaginative energy. The familiar midafternoon fatigue goes away; you may not even need to sleep much at night. Once you've lost the daily ritual of three meals, every moment becomes much the same as every other: pristine, vivid, and unburdened by the thickheadedness of the earth.

However, you don't have to fast to feel this way. The average raw foods follower can cultivate considerable lightness on fruits, vegetables, nuts, and raw grains. But there is a progression. Eating only fruits and vegetables makes you feel even lighter, and consuming nothing but fruit even more so. This is named fruitarianism, and it can be quite exhilarating.

There's something perfect about fruit. You can sit and hold an apple meditatively in your hand and stare at it and study its color. Fruit seems to glow when you pay close attention. It radiates. If you eat nothing but fruit, you begin to feel like the white flesh of a crisp apple: unblemished, even in consistency, drenched with life.

Of course, there's not a lot of protein in fruit, so it's possible to become malnourished on a fruitarian diet after a while. But it's not as bad as the final frontier for a raw foodist: breatharianism.

Breatharians claim to live on breath or energy alone. In her book *Living on Light: A Source of Nutrition for the New Millennium* (Koha Publishing, 1998), author Jasmuheen (that's her whole name) claims to have eaten no food at all for many years.

Breatharianism is hard to believe unless you have a religious faith in it, and indeed it has been traditionally associated with religious practices. Baba Hari Das, one of the teachers of Baba Ram Dass (Richard Alpert) claimed to live on nothing but one cup of milk a day for many years; he spoke of many other yogis who ate nothing at all.

Are these people faking? I've known of a few cases of breatharians caught sneaking food. One was a rather well known breatharian who was finally caught at McDonald's scarfing down a Big Mac at midnight.

But duplicity aside, there is another issue. Even to want to live only on air shows the rejectionist attitude implicit in raw foods: the notion that the right way to live is not to really be a person at all.

HUMAN OR NOT?

Most raw foods vegetarians do not become breatharian. They may fast for a while, but eventually they return to food. Eating fruit alone keeps the feeling of emptiness and transparency intact. Raw vegetables don't bring you down to earth very much either. But as soon as you add grains back in, even raw grains, the heaviness of life on earth begins to return. You may feel sleepy again after lunch, and you certainly start to notice the presence of a human body again. Your stomach also feels full after a meal.

Like anorexics, orthorexics may become excruciatingly aware when food remaining in the stomach creates even the slightest bit of expansion. Every sensation of the muscles in the abdomen is received like an affront, like an accusation. "You have overeaten," an inner voice calls out, even if it's only one slice of bread. "Feel your leaden stomach. You're not empty. You are heavy." You wait impatiently for the moment, some hours later, when that food has been digested and you feel light again. During the period when there is an indisputable sensation of having food in the body, you take vows never to eat heavy food again. You will stick, from then on, to fruit only.

In the spirituality known as Sufism, mystics speak of "angelic souls," individuals who wish to live as angels although they are on earth. Angelic souls have never quite accepted arriving here. It's heavier, thicker, and dirtier here than in the heavenly realms; where the angels live everything is pure and lucent. The earth is a place of suffering and fatigue, the angelic plane one of boundless energy and spirit.

Unable to come to terms with the weightiness of human life, angelic souls constantly opt for a pseudo-angelic existence. In the past they might have joined a monastery; today they might avoid human company and spend all their time reading or watching old movies. Another choice is to get into illegal drugs—or to become a raw foodist.

Othorexics in search of lightness are opting for the world of the spirit over the world of humanity. Back to Eden, back past Eden to the place before birth, onward to the place after death where there are no bodies at all.

Behind this seemingly free choice, however, is usually some fear. There may be a history of child abuse or a lesser experience that nonetheless has made the body distasteful. For some reason or another, raw-foodists really don't wish to feel the presence of the body.

Actually, there's nothing entirely wrong with feeling a bit heavy and tired after eating. Animals typically sleep after eating; it's a natural way to enhance digestion. The desire to avoid all feelings of fatigue and heaviness, to live like a spirit rather than a person, is really the need to run away from something.

Ask yourself: What is so wrong with living a human life? Are you doing this out of a spiritual choice or because you are afraid? Has your body been hurt? Are you ashamed of yourself? Do you wish you didn't have a body at all?

In fact, we are people and not just spirits. Isn't there plenty of time to be disembodied after we die? Wouldn't it make sense to live out a human life while being human?

GRAPEFRUITS IN JANUARY?

Besides the way it hides fear of living a human life, there are other problems with raw-foodism, intellectual inconsistencies and weaknesses that proponents would like to ignore. For example, if the goal is to return to the natural state, does it really make sense to eat lettuce and grapefruit in January?

Unless you live in the tropics, lettuce and grapefruit don't grow in January. They have to be flown or trucked in, under refrigerated conditions. Is this natural? Did our ancestors have access to an international network of transportation? As we will see in the next chapter, the macrobiotic theory of diet explicitly focuses on locally grown produce, on the theory that if you live in Maine, food from Mexico might not even be good for you. Even if you don't accept macrobiotic philosophy, there certainly is something to think about in this objection.

There are other problems as well. Perhaps the most significant is that the Edenic state so earnestly desired by raw-foodists never existed: Anthropology tells us that our ancient ancestors ate plenty of meat along with their nuts and fruits. There was no historical period of pure vegetarianism. Think of the primal people that remain in the world: The Aborigines of Australia, the Bushmen of Africa, the natives of North and South America all ate meat and all cooked their food. If primal people have any wisdom, raw-foodism and even total vegetarianism do not; they are an invention of modern civilized people with time on their hands, who are yearning for a Golden Age and feel free to invent it out of their desires.

And from the point of view of modern nutrition there is one great additional flaw in raw foodism: It lacks any source of vitamin B12. You have to either take it in supplement form or eat B12-supplemented yeast. Can that be right? Can that be natural?

Raw food is definitely tasty. But is it really sensible to make it a way of life? Do you really always have to feel light, empty, and transparent? I'd recommend instead living as a human being on this earth and eating a balanced diet that also includes a great deal of raw food.

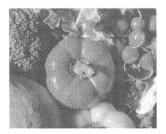

8.

Macrobiotics

As described in the last chapter, raw foods theory seeks a return to the Natural State imagined to exist prior to civilization. Never mind that no such state ever existed; the dream is to undo time and return to the historical womb. Raw-foodism fits well both into the ascetic tradition of Western civilization and the romantic longing for the Natural State. Sin and redemption combine with the yearning to find answers in one fell swoop of radical reconstruction to create a theory that is rejectionistic, simple, and oriented toward a precivilized state.

Macrobiotics, on the other hand, arises out of a civilization whose ideals tend toward refining civilized life rather than rejecting it. In the Asian cultures of China, Korea, and Japan, the goal of most forms of spirituality was to find a way to live graciously in the world, not to reject it. The raw craving for perfection in an imagined Natural State is replaced by an acceptance of the reality that we live with other people in a complex and sophisticated society that bears very little relationship to the world of our hunter-gatherer ancestors.

Rather than suggest that we should overthrow all the institutions of modern life, from the cooking stove on up, Asian philosophy tends toward practical suggestions that make modern life more livable. Practicing tai chi every day, for example, is consistent with life in the big city; it doesn't involve giving up everything and hiking twenty miles a day. It is a stylized, elaborate adaptation to culture from a part of the world that has had a high culture for many thousands of years and does not to any extent whatsoever idealize the precivilized Natural State.

In diet this philosophical orientation has led to the development of a variety of related approaches aimed more at achieving balance than at stripping away. Where raw foods theory talks about cleansing, diets originating in classical Asian medicine talk about balancing. Raw foods theory looks on the world of foods and sees good and evil; this approach sees neither good nor evil but rather foods that can be either healthy or unhealthy depending on how they are used. Raw foods theory seeks an extreme, while traditional Asian diets seek moderation.

According to the medical theories that originated in ancient China and spread to other Asian countries, each food possesses a quality, or energy, that makes it appropriate for those people who need it and unhealthy for those who do not. If you are deficient in the energy that, say, chicken contains, eating chicken (in moderation) will help you. If you eat either too much or too little chicken, however, the net effect will be harmful. And if you are not deficient in that energy, even a little chicken will be bad for you. Perhaps in the last case you need more vegetables or even a specific vegetable.

Theoretically, at least, it's not that certain foods are good and others bad but that they must be eaten in a proper balance. Indeed, it is errors in balance rather than the specific foods that make a diet unhealthy.

Actually, there is one bad food in Asian dietary philosophy, one dietary element believed to sap health and cause disease: raw foods! You don't find salad in traditional Chinese restaurants, because it's believed to cause arthritis, cancer, and numerous other diseases. Another blow against the consistency of dietary theories!

Aside from the evil of rawness, most other foods have a place for the right person at the right time. Once acquainted with the Asian approach it's hard not to see raw-foodism as simplistic, naïve, and rather American; a "one size fits all" solution that recognizes no individual variation. Can one diet really be good for everyone? Probably not. Asian dietary theory implicitly recognizes this, and whether or not it has the details right, the general concept is difficult to argue with.

In the West macrobiotics is the best-known version of traditional Asian dietary philosophy. Originated by George Ohsawa and popularized by Michio Kushi, it became enormously influential in the United States. Its following in America seems to have decreased in recent years, but it remains the most prominent form of Eastern dietary thought in America.

Macrobiotics is also one of the most likely dietary approaches to create orthorexia. It draws the mind into an obsession in a sophisticated way. What it satisfies in particular is the yearning to have everything under strict control.

YIN AND YANG

The concept behind macrobiotics is much simpler than other traditional dietary philosophies from Asia. It leaves out much detail involving each organ of the body and focuses almost entirely on the classic Taoist principle of yin and yang, the notion that the universe is made up of opposites.

Yang is male, yin is female; yang is heaven, yin is earth; yang is contraction, yin is expansion; yang is power, yin is receptivity; yang is dry, yin is damp; yang is hot, yin is cold; yang is hard, yin is fragile; etc. Using this metaphoric framework is a rich enterprise.

According to macrobiotic theorists, we naturally, unconsciously, seek a balance of yin and yang in our diets. Thus the Western diet, which contains many yang foods (meat, cheese, refined salt), causes us to crave extremely yin foods (sweets, salads, ice cream) and to need many medications (which are also yin).

But when you eat macrobiotically, you attempt to stay in the middle, between yin and yang, and avoid the extremes. Foods in the balanced category are supposed to make up the staple of diet. However, even within that category it is important to balance the opposites.

For example, a carrot is more yang than a purple cabbage. Food can also be altered by cooking. Increasing the length of cooking, as well as the temperature and pressure, adds a yang element, as does adding salt or other seasoning. The reverse increases the yin aspect of diet. According to classic macrobiotic thinking, the most perfect of all foods is brown rice. In itself it is a balance between yin and yang: the spreading, yin forces of the ripening grain against the contractive, yang impulse of the husk.

The exact way you should eat depends also on environmental

factors. As Kushi explains, "When we plan our menus in the warmer season of the year or in a warmer environment, it is safer to balance these yang climatic factors with slightly more foods from the yin category. Conversely, when selecting foods in the colder season of the year or in colder regions, we can offset these yin environmental factors with a diet slightly higher in food from the yang category."

This means that more root vegetables are eaten in the winter and autumn, and more leafy green vegetables in the hotter times of the year. Grains should be balanced by the season, too: Long-grain rice is more yin and should be eaten during the hotter time of year; short-grain rice is yang and therefore better eaten during the cold months. Certain lifestyles, too, dictate the choice of diet. The more physically active you are, the lower the proportion of grains you should have in your diet, while those engaged in intensive mental or spiritual exercises need to increase the amount of grains consumed.

Another beautiful aspect of macrobiotic theory is the concept that nature tends to seek balance in all its parts. Therefore, the foods that grow naturally in a particular area, or at a particular time of year, contain elements that can automatically balance other factors in the environment. Vegetables that keep throughout the winter—such as winter squash, pumpkin and root vegetables—are thought to help balance the cold of the winter with its yang inner heat; a winter squash is thought to have stored up a tremendous amount of heat over the many months it took to grow. Similarly, the fruits that grow so abundantly in hot climates are yin and thought to contain a coolness that balances that heat.

Macrobiotics, therefore, argues against eating foods imported long distances, thought to lack the balancing properties of local, in-season produce. (For an exception, see below.) Grapefruits grown in

Florida and intemperately consumed in the North Dakota winter would be thought altogether unhealthy; whereas they balance the heat in Florida, they exacerbate the cold of North Dakota, leading to "cold illnesses" such as arthritis. A macrobiotic devotee is supposed to focus his dietary attention on in-season, local produce.

The very complexity of the macrobiotic diet, its innumerable nuances, make up a great part of its attraction. It's possible to become quite absorbed with calculations and balancing, tuning your diet like an orchestra and paying a great deal of attention to interesting matters of environment and lifestyle choice. This is one of the ways in which macrobiotics can so easily lead to orthorexia. The very complexity of the theory makes it seductive and absorbing, setting the stage for obsession. When you follow the theory to a tee, you have to weigh and measure everything you eat and drink; even vegetables have to be sliced in just the right way. It makes a huge difference whether you toast your sesame seeds and for how long, because doing so increases their yang potential; there is no innocence in cooking at all.

MACROBIOTICS VERSUS RAW FOODS

Beyond their direct contradiction regarding rawness, there is a strong emotional difference between raw foods an macrobiotics. You can see this clearly in the definition of a fast in each system. Raw-foodists think of fasts as eating next to nothing at all. For a macrobiotic adherent, to fast means to eat nothing but brown rice. Compare the effect of this to the otherworldly impulses of a raw-foodist, and the difference should be clear. When you fast on water, you become transparent; when you eat brown rice, you may mortify your gustatory desires, but you do not float away. The diet is more boring than productive of an altered state. Macrobiotics leads to people who are grounded. They do not float around at the treetops, plucking ripe fruit out of the luminous atmosphere; they eat bowls of rice and feel full. They plan carefully, they are weighty, they are practical. Macrobiotics is to raw-foodism as a brick is to a balloon; it is much more deliberate, grounded, civilized. Nonetheless, as we shall see, it is just as likely to promote orthorexia.

BEYOND HEALTH

There is no question that the philosophy of yin and yang can enrich and deepen your view of life as a whole. One of the unique and impressive outcomes of this philosophy is that you are less likely to take sides.

Classically, yin and yang need each other to be complete; the goal is balance, not extremism. From this perspective, for example, Democrats and Republicans might be seen as two halves of a coin rather than distinct choices, one right and the other wrong. (Perhaps there are more Taoists in the U.S. electorate than one might imagine, since it seems to be the fervent hope of many to elect a President of one party and a congressional majority of the other, so neither side will posses too much power.) This is a part of philosophical Taoism, and like any other philosophical approach, it can reward study with a deepening understanding of some of the nuances of being alive.

Macrobiotic adherents do tend to cultivate a yin/yang view of the world, something that it is hard to fault. However, the theory goes a bit far when it suggests that yin/yang balancing of food will solve your personal problems, as well as the world's.

The following passage from Michio and Aveline Kushi's *Macrobiotic Diet* (Japan Publications, 1993) shows that the founders of this approach are just as enlarged in their view of the meaning of their diet as are any raw-foodists: "The biological and spiritual reconstruction of humanity begins with . . . returning to a way of eating more in harmony with the environment. . . . [D]iet is *the* [emphasis mine] crucial factor in determining and shaping physical health, psychological character and social behavior."

A large claim indeed, much like the conclusion that cooking food is the primary enemy of mankind.

"Needless to say, there are many factors other than dietary habits which influence human destiny," Michio Kushi generously allows, "but among all of them, dietary habits in relation to natural climatic conditions is the primary factor, directing, motivating and reciprocally interacting with other factors."

The goal is not only personal happiness, but also world peace: "Without correcting individual dietary habits, personal health and happiness will not be achieved, and without correcting society's dietary habits, environmental harmony and global peace will not be realized."

BUT IS IT TRUE?

The philosophy behind macrobiotics is genuinely interesting, possesses an internal logic, and can cause one to rethink some of one's assumptions. If it makes sense and is profound, it must be right; that's how it feels.

But just because something makes sense, that doesn't mean it's true. I believe that Descartes first enunciated this principle. Any intellectually satisfying theory carries an emotional conviction of authenticity. This sensation of truth has nothing to do with actual truth; the most tear-jerkingly romantic of Hollywood movies feels true at the time we see it because we want it to be true, but life still doesn't really work that way. Similarly, a dietary philosophy that ties together many loose ends will carry an automatic cachet of universal truth regardless of whether it is true.

And if you look at it closely, macrobiotics has some genuine problems. Perhaps the most glaring is its focus on Japanese foods. For some coincidental reason, in this Japanese-derived theory many Japanese-derived foods are best—even if they are neither local nor in season. Umeboshi plums (actually a pickled Japanese apricot) are one example, thought to purify the body and heal wounds, and highly praised by macrobiotic theorists. But umeboshi is grown and made in Japan, not in Boston or Texas. This recommendation doesn't exactly fit with the profound theory of macrobiotics. It's simply an ethnic preference.

The same goes for the superiority of rice over wheat (they don't eat much wheat in Japan), adzuki beans over pinto beans, and sea vegetables over zucchini (the latter being a quintessential locally grown and derived produce in the United States, the former a staple of Japanese diet). Miso soup, kombu, tamari, natto, burdock, tofu, tempeh—a hundred other Japanese culinary preferences are assigned a mysteriously high place in the macrobiotic pantheon of foods. This isn't a philosophical orientation; it's what Michio Kushi grew up eating and believes we should all eat, too.

A much bigger problem is whether or not all the weighing, measuring, and balancing that goes into macrobiotics really makes a difference. Admittedly, looked at from afar, macrobiotics is simply a non-dairy vegetarianism. This is undoubtedly a very healthy approach to diet, provided you get enough protein and take vitamin B12 supplements. (It is nearly impossible to get enough vitamin B12 from plant sources of food.) But beyond this, does the detail of macrobiotics, the detailed balancing of yin and yang in foods, make any difference? Is there any real reason to think about all this stuff?

Regardless of the many testimonials and theoretical explanations macrobiotic pioneers cite, there is certainly no proof that eating macrobiotically is any better than consuming a balanced non-dairy vegetarian diet. The testimonials actually don't mean a thing; there are just as many testimonials for dietary theories that contradict macrobiotics in one or more essential principles. And all the cosmic reasoning in the world about human evolution and the principles of the ordering of the universe doesn't show that the theory is true; it just impresses the mind.

Not only all this, but keep in mind also that macrobiotics is not actually an ancient philosophy; it is a creation of George Ohsawa, who believed that eating only brown rice was the highest path in life. The ancient Asian traditions out of which macrobiotics originated are nowhere near so strict; they follow some of the same principles but don't get into the same compulsive detail.

THE HIDDEN AGENDA OF MACROBIOTICS

It is no accident that macrobiotics is so strict. In fact, strictness is its underlying emotional agenda. People are attracted to macrobiotics because they want to gain greater control over themselves. By managing food down to the minutest details, they imagine that they are managing their lives as minutely. The sense of mastery in the food arena provides a feel of power over everything.

However, as described in Chapter 5, you can't really control your life so perfectly, you can only pretend to do so. Not only that, the very attempt can make you a little bit crazy.

The tale of a man I shall call Carl shows the macrobiotic obsession over control. The story went that he'd once been severely emotionally ill but that he'd cured himself by taking up macrobiotics. After I met him, I thought perhaps I'd describe his history a bit differently: He's compensated for his psychosis by taking up a life of ritual almost as complex as that of an autistic.

When we met for lunch at a macrobiotic café, he unconsciously rearranged all the items on the table to fit in a geometric pattern. His speech was filled with allusions to regularity and order and obsession with food, and his movement and features were so angular and stylized that no one could mistake him for a healthy person, even at fifty paces.

But in those days Carl was often presented as an example of the healing power of macrobiotics! He had been interviewed in macrobiotic magazines and showcased at macrobiotic conventions. I didn't think he was healed; he had just found a way to compensate for his interior chaos. That he could function at all in life was a tribute not to his diet but to his substitution of dietary obsession for a less orderly form of madness.

Still, Carl was living a pretty good life, and a much better one than you might expect, given his illness. I can't fault him, and he has every right to be grateful to macrobiotics for giving him the structure that he needs to get by. But it can get much worse than this. Whenever I think of macrobiotics today, I remember Michael and Jerry, a father and son. This story embodies the dark side of macrobiotics, the way in which obsessiveness and control are not always innocent.

Jerry wasn't the patient, but I was more worried about him than about his father. Michael came to me wanting assistance for his frequent headaches. He had been seeing a colleague of mine, an acupuncturist, but hadn't found relief. He thought I might be able to help him.

Michael was tall and thin, and he wore the facial expression so common among followers of macrobiotics. It's hard to describe. The skin looks slightly darker than usual; it's tight, without any hanging folds or obvious smile lines. The shape of the face itself seems different, too, perhaps again due to the tightness of the skin. It's more angular, more like a polygon than a circle or an oval. If you know anyone who has diligently practiced macrobiotics for a while, you'll know what I mean.

Michael spoke to me in a slow, measured voice about the time of day when his head would begin to throb and about the foods and environmental factors that seemed to trigger it (splurging on large red beans rather than adzuki beans, was, as I recall, a guilty habit he felt free to admit to me). But I couldn't stop looking at Jerry.

He, too, wore the macro face, but it was more than that. He looked sick. He leaned idly against his father's chair and stared at nothing. Although Jerry was about four years old, there was nothing of the mischief and curiosity I'd expect at that age. Instead of rampaging around the room opening my drawers and scattering the tongue depressors far and wide, like a normal four-year-old, he just leaned against his father's chair. He didn't even tap his feet or pull on his father's arm. His skin didn't look right either. Something about it reminded me of another child, but I couldn't place the recollection.

Michael went on at length monotonously, reciting types of grains and their association with the parts of his head that would subsequently hurt. "Millet grown in the United States gives me a headache in my left temple, while millet imported from Asia makes my neck hurt. Now, isn't that interesting?" There was no more expression in that last observation than you would expect to hear in the voice of someone reading off a charge-card number.

Finally Jerry moved. He took the fingers of his right hand and pulled up some of the skin off the back of his left hand. The skin came up in a little tent, and when he let go it, held its shape for a while.

Tenting! That was it. I'd last seen it in a child brought in to intensive care after a week of severe vomiting and diarrhea. It was a classic sign of significant dehydration.

"How much fluid do you drink?" I suddenly asked the dad.

He looked guiltily at me. "Sometimes as much as six ounces a day."

Had I not been used to macrobiotic adherents, I would have thought he was embarrassed about drinking too little water. But I knew that macrobiotics counsels restriction of fluid intake in many circumstances. He thought he was drinking too much!

This is different from most other schools of natural medicine. Dating back to the day when the kidney was thought to need regular flushing (as if it were a toilet), naturopathic medicine has decided that you should drink eight glasses of water daily. This theory has so taken hold that you will read it in many places as standard medical advice for optimal health. Actually, there is no particular foundation to the "lots of water" theory either. Personally, I think that it is best to drink when you're thirsty and stop drinking when you're not thirsty anymore. The body should be able to tell whether it is short on water or not.

But macrobiotics, in its ascetic wisdom, takes the opposite tack of naturopathy and believes that less is more. Even in the fiercely dry climate of summertime Fort Collins, Colorado, Michael felt that he should drink less than six ounces of liquid a day.

And what was he asking of his child?

"Are you pretty good at monitoring your son's water intake?" I asked, trying to phrase my question positively.

The father brightened up. "Absolutely. We make sure he does the right thing. Three ounces of water a day, measured out. No exceptions. I don't let him cheat the way I do."

I shuddered inwardly. Making an excuse, I stepped out of my office, and called his former acupuncturist.

"Diane, I have this fellow Michael in my office," I said.

"Michael? With the kid? Steven, hold him there and I'll call Child Protective Services. He bolted this morning when I confronted him about it, and the phone number and address he gave me are wrong."

Just then Michael came out of the room, holding his son. "Anything, wrong?" he asked. "Maybe I should go."

I put down the phone and thought fast. I would never be able to hold him long enough for CPS. If he left, who knows what would happen? Should I dial 911 and have the police chase him down? What if he got away? Maybe a less violent strategy would work better.

"Actually, I was just calling up a macrobiotic practitioner," I lied. I walked with him back to the treatment room.

"I think I've found the problem," I said. "You're neglecting to take into account the local balance of yin and yang."

"How do you mean?"

"In Japan, or in Boston, the weather is humid. It makes sense to counteract that yin tendency with a yang restriction on dietary fluid. But here the weather is very yang. Plants don't puff up—they shrink to the ground. The proper quest for balance would suggest a much higher water intake—much higher."

"How much?" he said, both suspiciously and, I thought, longingly.

I scribbled some fake calculations on a piece of paper. "How much do you weigh?" I asked, and then I followed it up with other queries about him and his son.

Finally I came up with two figures. "Six cups a day for you and four cups a day for Jerry. "But that's just an approximation," I said. "You should probably drink when you're thirsty. You can trust your body to seek the necessary balance."

Suddenly Jerry lit up. "Can I have drink from the water cooler?"

"I don't know," Michael said. "I'm not sure if your mother would like it."

"Have her give me a call, and I'll calculate her optimum intake as well."

Michael still hesitated, and then brightened. "I think that what you say makes sense. Come on, son, let's drink water."

They walked out together to the water cooler on their expedition, their shared indulgence, like father and son going out skiing, skydiving, or mountain-biking together for the first time. Watching them drink, I felt as if I were tasting water for the first time myself. I thought I could almost see the little boy's blood begin to flow again, his skin grow soft and elastic.

Later, the acupuncturist and I decided that we were legally obligated to call Child Protective Services anyway. The home visit found no problems. Michael and his wife were good parents; they had just been seduced by the crazy logic of orthorexia.

Besides dehydration, the most common physical health problem I have seen with macrobiotics is vitamin B12 deficiency. This is not caused by macrobiotics' specific details but simply by the fact that it is a form of non-dairy vegetarianism (or vegan diet). No known native peoples have ever been vegan. That there's basically no way to get enough of this essential vitamin without eating at least a bit of animal products is an indication that it isn't really a healthy approach to diet.

But macrobiotics supplemented with vitamin B12, and carried through sensibly enough to allow enough water to live on, is a healthy diet. Eating predominantly whole grains, vegetables, and soy products will probably reduce the risk of cancer, heart disease, and other major illnesses dramatically in later life. Here, as with most forms of orthorexia, the risk is not so much physical as it is emotional and spiritual.

Macrobiotics is such a comprehensive form of kitchen spirituality that it almost inevitably takes over the entire soul of the individual who has fallen into it. It fascinates with its philosophy, difficulty, and seeming deep wisdom; it turns the kitchen into a shrine and eating into the most sacred act of life; it makes control the defining principle of life and rigidity the nature of worship. It kills the spontaneity of life and absorbs its poetry into a mass of rules and restrictions.

If you are trapped in the rulism of macrobiotics, the structure worship, the miserly measuring out of food in grams and half grams, the parsing out of the day and the seasons with a yardstick made of root vegetables, the counting of the minutes in grains of short grain brown rice, the reduction of the world itself to a ricy flavor, the slow and thoughtful chewing of vegetables and beans while the world goes on riotously about you, the living in a web of imagined safety created by strictly controlled edibles—if any of this out-of-control controlism describes you, read the story I tell in Chapter 16 of a woman who escaped from macrobiotics. You may be much happier for it.

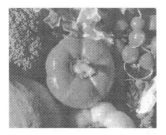

9.

The Zone

While macrobiotics fascinates by its complexity, the Zone diet grabs the mind because its premise contradicts accepted medical wisdom. While medical authorities have been telling us for years that complex carbohydrates such as grains should be the mainstay of our diets, the Zone diet suggests that we should eat practically no carbohydrates at all.

Although other dietary theories (such as Protein Power and the Atkins diet) espouse similar principles, the Zone diet has become the most influential of these approaches, spawning an industry of Zone power bars, Zone Web sites, and Zone support groups. Barry Sears, this theory's founder, claims that eating "in the Zone" will not only help you lose weight but will prolong life, prevent illness, enhance sexual vitality, improve skin tone, increase brain function, and basically provide every healing wonder you can imagine.

In actual fact, the theory behind the Zone diet is intriguing, and it might have considerable truth to it. However, it can also become a direct route to orthorexia. Before I go into any details, I'd like to return to an older concept, hypoglycemia.

BEFORE THE ZONE: HYPOGLYCEMIA

Back in the 1970s and '80s hypoglycemia was the biggest dietary buzzword (as big as candida was in the early nineties and as the blood type theory seems destined to become in the new millennium). I first heard about it from Brian, one of my college roommates and friends. Since about age fifteen Brian had experienced fatigue and drowsiness as constant companions. No matter whether he slept well or not, no matter whether he exercised or not, a thick fog enveloped his mind and invisible weights held down his body. "I don't have any initiative," he'd say. "It's all dull in here." Brian also suffered from headaches, mental confusion, blurred vision, and sensitivity to certain patterns of bricks on the ground.

In his first year of college the symptoms became so bad that he finally sought medical assistance. A comprehensive medical workup led to no diagnosis other than "You're fine. It must be all in your head." Brian was not willing to accept this explanation, and like so many other people, he went straight from the doctors who could not help to the books that claimed they could.

After a brief run through B vitamins, chlorophyll, and ascorbic acid (popular alternative therapies for fatigue at the time), Brian discovered the theory of hypoglycemia. The book he read (I can't remember which one it was among the legion of antisugar tomes) seemed to describe him exactly. It explained the way our bodies manage blood-sugar levels and the reaction that happens when we consume sweet foods. First our blood sugar rises; next insulin flows out from the pancreas; finally, in response, blood-sugar levels fall to normal. According to the theory of hypoglycemia, however, in some people this natural regulatory process overshoots its mark, dropping blood-sugar levels past normal to subnormal, causing a state of low blood sugar ("hypo" meaning "low," "glycemia" meaning "blood-sugar level").

It is a fact that the brain depends on circulating sugar (as glucose) for its energy. Therefore, the theory states, this lack of adequate sugar in the blood can impair the function of the brain, leading to confusion, dullness, fatigue, and all of Brian's other symptoms as well. Furthermore, as the body frantically attempts to raise blood-sugar levels, it releases a flood of hormones, including adrenaline. These create the typical sensations of anxiety, sweating, and craving for sugar.

Hypoglycemic people often feel a need to eat sweets an hour or so after eating; however, if they give in, the result will be another roller-coaster ride up and down the blood-sugar track. Instead of sweet foods Brian's book recommended frequent small meals, but none of them high in sugary or starchy foods. It proposed that hypoglycemic people should concentrate instead on vegetables and protein (Zone dieters will recognize the similarity).

For Brian, protein meant a thick steak. He started skipping the food-service meals at college (no great loss!) and instead dined on fat T-bones he cooked over a forbidden burner in our dorm room. It helped him a lot. Although he never became truly energetic, he found he had much longer periods during the day when his mind functioned clearly and he felt a sense of energy.

By the time I became a practicing alternative medicine physician in the mid-eighties, hypoglycemia was going out of fashion, but at its peak millions of people explained their fatigue and other symptoms by invoking it. There's no doubt, of course, that some people have attacks of sweatiness and anxiety when the last eaten food runs out. I do myself. But there is one major problem with the hypoglycemia theory: It turns out that these symptoms don't correlate very well with actual blood-sugar levels. When a hypoglycemic is sweating and yearning for food, his or her blood sugar isn't particularly low; in fact, people without hypoglycemic symptoms may regularly have much lower blood-sugar levels.

Thus, "hypoglycemia" doesn't actually involve hypoglycemia! True hypoglycemia occurs almost exclusively in people with diabetes, when they take too high a dose of diabetes medications. Rather, in what is called "hypoglycemia," the body is behaving as if blood-sugar levels were terribly low, even though they are not. We don't know why or how this occurs.

However, even if the theory of hypoglycemia is wrong, the treatment sometimes works. As a physician I have encountered numerous people who felt better when they relinquished all sugary and starchy foods and switched over to a high-protein or high-fat diet. Why should this help when blood-sugar levels aren't even low in the first place?

Over subsequent years new explanations came into vogue. First it was candida, and the theory that sugar feeds yeast (see Chapter 10); later a resurgence of food allergy theory claimed it was allergies to wheat and other grains that caused the problem. The latest explanation comes from the Zone diet.

ZONING

Barry Sears had the inspiration to turn the old hypoglycemia concept upside down. Instead of focusing on blood-sugar levels, he decided to focus at the other side of the equation: insulin release.

As I mentioned earlier, when you eat starchy foods, your body has to release insulin to help you process it. According to Sears, it is excessive insulin levels rather than low blood-sugar levels that cause the problems. His books emphasize controlling insulin levels as the way to reduce fatigue and other symptoms of "hypoglycemia." He also believes that high insulin levels cause weight gain, and ultimately increased heart disease and early death.

He may be onto something here. A considerable body of evidence does suggest that high insulin levels (so-called pre-diabetes), can play a significant role in heart disease. Sears marshals this evidence, along with interesting reasoning about the ancestral diet of humans (cavemen ate little starch), and combines it with research of his own to create a provocative theory.

However, at the present time the Zone diet can't be regarded as proven. Much of Sears's reasoning is still pretty speculative and his evidence less convincing than he makes it sound. For example, he cites studies in which diabetics switched to a Zone diet and their blood-sugar control improved. However, it's a well-known fact that if you enroll people in a study, their condition is almost guaranteed to improve, if for no other reason than that they pay closer attention to self-care. (This is called the "study effect.") Also, he has a habit of exaggerating how well we understand the function of various hormones and substances in the body. For example, his discussion of serotonin in *The Anti-Aging Zone* (Regan Books, 1999) goes far beyond what scientists really know. He makes it seem that low serotonin means depression, but the real picture is far more complex and murkier.

Most important of all, there's no direct evidence that the Zone diet helps you live longer. Only the Mediterranean diet can claim any significant evidence in that regard, and it includes over

50 percent whole grains. (It also involves a high intake of tomatoes, rich in potentially life-extending lycopenes; other fresh vegetables, high in numerous natural antioxidants; and the beneficial essential fatty acids found in olive or canola oil.) Sears thinks that the Zone diet will work even better, but we don't really know this. Still, it is perfectly reasonable to get excited about an intriguing possibility like the Zone diet, and give it a go.

THE ORTHOREXIC ZONE

There is a difference here, as always, between following a diet and becoming an orthorexic. The basic diet as outlined by Barry Sears is not obsessive in character. He very deliberately recommends a relaxed approach to eating and outlines numerous steps for making Zone dieting quite easy and graceful. But that doesn't seem to be the way his followers take it. Too frequently this rather elegant and tasty dietary theory crosses the line into obsession.

There are Web sites devoted to people who Zone, and a quick look at the posted messages reveals the familiar pattern of dietary obsession. For many people Zoning has become a way of life, a profound obsession over dietary principles. The sequential letters reveal constant struggle with temptation, guilt, and fear over breaking the rules, and penitent returns to the holy way of Zone.

Orthorexic Zoners spend much of their day talking about their diet and debating the fine points of the theory like Talmudic scholars, using the works of Barry Sears as scripture. There's an obvious desperation underlying many posted notes, a panic over straying off the true path, and a mortal fear of lusting after the foreign gods of muffins and toast.

Much of this is similar to what happens with all other dietary theories when they are taken to excess. But the Zone seems to have a particular focus: the search for immortality. Much of the desperation behind the writings of committed Zoners is the hope that by taking desperate and rigid control of food, they can cheat death.

THE SEARCH FOR IMMORTALITY

I will not be thought radical, I trust, if I point out that we are all going to die, although I might be thought impolite to bring up the subject. Death is lurking; it is going to get you and me and everyone else. Everything we dream for, pursue, build, and create is going to vanish when the cells of our bodies expire. As one Zen writer put it, "Life is a boat that you take out into the ocean for a while, and then it sinks." But for obvious reasons we have a great desire to postpone the event and even to pretend it isn't ever going to happen.

Because it claims so much in the way of anti-aging powers, the Zone diet strongly activates this desire to cheat death. It is easy to discern behind the desperate postings of the more extreme Zoners a horror and terror at the prospect that their lives will end someday. Fueling their obsessive food behavior is the passionate desire to hide the face of death under a pile of high-protein snacks with low-glycemic-index vegetables, laced with omega-3 fatty acids.

Therapist David Knight posted one of my orthorexia articles on a Zone site, and the response was both troubling and exciting. Predictably, a few people thought that I was persecuting them, cruelly criticizing their diet choices. One letter suggested that I might be an agent of the wheat industry. But other correspondents thought that the concept was worth thinking about. As one person replied (I'm paraphrasing and combining stories to some extent), "I believe that having a certain level of obsession with food is normal. Keep in mind that we need food to live. . . . However, my eating habits have become such that my whole life is controlled by this obsession, not just my eating-related life. I think I have to admit that it's a real problem for me. To be fair to all of us, it's certainly normal to become diet-obsessed at the start of a new way of eating, whether it is the Zone diet or something else. But I've been doing it for years, and still spend all my time calculating the protein grams in my next meal. I wish I could relax about it. I realize now that I hate feeling obsessed this way."

Another writer's story is more poignant: "After reading Bratman's piece, I realize I've got the disease he's talking about. I've got orthorexia. Actually, I'm practically crazy with it. I don't think I've gone a waking minute without thinking about food for five years. I am no longer dieting to fix a problem. The diet now is the problem."

But it can get more extreme than the Zone.

THE CAVEMAN DIET

Just as raw foods vegetarianism can go to an extreme and become fruitarianism, the Zone diet can crawl inexorably onward to become the Caveman or Paleolithic diet. Some of the theoretical underpinnings of the Zone diet invoke the food eaten by our ancestors prior to the invention of agriculture. Sears quite correctly points out that our genetics haven't changed since those days. It's a fact that a hundred thousand years simply isn't long enough for much genetic progression in a species whose generations are twenty years apart. However, in that brief time (from a biological point of view) our diet has taken a 180-degree turn. We turned from eating mostly meat and wild plants to a diet focused primarily on grains. The Zone diet turns back the clock. In theory the Zone diet should bring us closer to the food we were genetically programmed to accept.

The Caveman (or Paleolithic) diet takes this logic a further step and suggests that we not only renounce grains but eat as much as possible as Cavemen did. As described by Ray Audette in *NEANDERTHIN A Caveman's Guide to Nutrition*, this approach involves trying to eat like a primeval hunter-gatherer. Weeds ripped out of a nearby wetland and scarfed raw like salad would, if eaten along with fresh deer (and mammoth, if available), most closely simulate our genetically programmed dietary habits. Certain compromises are necessitated by the lack of wild game in most urban settings, but the goal is clear: to imitate as closely as possible the food our ancestors turned to when they first came down from the trees. This primarily means meat and raw fruits and vegetables. As the coinage "Neanderthin" indicates, much of this approach is also driven by the desire to lose weight.

The Caveman diet has some spiritual similarities to raw foods theory. After all, it consists mostly of raw foods, and the longing to return to the Natural State informs both eating plans. The one big difference between the two approaches is, of course, the inclusion of meat in the diet. Anthropologically, the Caveman approach is more accurate, since our human and nonhuman ancestors did indeed eat meat, but it leads to a very different psychological state. While raw-foodists cultivate the transparent, angelic, luminous state, Cavemen dieters are a more earthy, "spear in hand" sort of community.

TO ZONE OR NOT TO ZONE

Returning from these extremes to the Zone diet itself, the question naturally arises whether it is a sensible diet to follow. The answer is, there's no way to know. Barry Sears's arguments are intriguing but far from watertight. You can certainly try his method to see whether you feel better (or lose weight) in the short run; however, whether it will actually make you live longer remains to be seen. Of course, you only have one life in which to try a lifelong diet. If the Zone diet turns out not to prolong your life, you won't be able to go back and try something else! Consider yourself part of an experiment for later generations.

But whatever you do, try to do it without getting obsessed. Think of Zoning like brushing your teeth, rather than like propitiating the health gods to ensure long life.

If it is too late, and you are already obsessed with life in the Zone, see Section 3 for what you can do to break free.

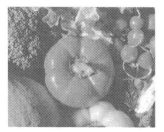

10.

Candida and Other Simple Solutions

Thankfully it's now begun to fade away, but in the early nineties it was nearly impossible to walk into the office of an alternative practitioner without receiving the diagnosis of Candida. Properly called "Yeast Hypersensitivity syndrome," this pseudodisease also went by the completely incorrect name of "systemic candidiasis." It was the successor to hypoglycemia, and a fad disease that is now, mercifully, beginning to fade from the scene.

Introduced by Orion Truss and popularized by William Crook, the candida theory clearly has a kernel of truth to it. In its most reasonable form, the concept can be stated as follows: Some people form too much yeast in the body and subsequently develop an allergy to it.

Candida is short for *Candida albicans,* the ubiquitous yeast that causes diaper rash, vaginal yeast infections, and, occasionally, thrush. There is no way to eliminate all the candida in and on your body, because it lives there naturally. But certain influences can cause *C.*

albicans to proliferate out of control, causing annoying but seldom dangerous symptoms.

The most common cause of excess candida is the use of antibiotics, which, by killing the bacteria that are its natural enemies, allow the yeast to proliferate. This is why many women reliably develop vaginal yeast infections following a course of ampicillin or other broad-spectrum antibiotic, and why many physicians prescribe three to seven anti-yeast suppositories right along with the use of the antibiotic prescription. The friendly bacterium *Lactobacillus acidophilus* also competes with candida for real estate. For this reason, yogurt douches and oral consumption of acidophilus tablets can help prevent antibiotic-related yeast infections.

Excessive growth of candida in the vagina, mouth, or elsewhere causes discomfort, itching, and a white discharge. However, in his 1983 book *The Missing Diagnosis*, Orion Truss proposed another consequence that he thought occurred fairly frequently but went unrecognized: yeast hypersensitivity. He reasoned that excessive candida could give rise to a candida allergy. The symptoms would be very similar to those of food allergies, but since yeast actually lives in your body, unlike allergenic foods, these symptoms might become more constant and severe. Truss suggested that many common symptoms might be due to yeast hypersensitivity, including headaches, fatigue, muscle pain, and frequent sinus infections.

It's a reasonable idea. Considering that the widespread use of antibiotics has undoubtedly given more people excessive yeast than ever before in history, there have been plenty of opportunities for yeast allergies to develop. However, is it really a widespread disease? Judging by the way the diagnosis has gone out of fashion, I rather doubt it.

It was William Crook who propelled Truss's idea into the popular consciousness. His *Yeast Connection* was followed by numerous volumes for specific audiences, all selling the idea that Candida (the syndrome) was one of the greatest epidemics of the century. Perhaps the greatest selling point of Crook's books was that he made up a difficult diet, and one that he said could cure many common health problems. Soon he had the forces of orthorexia on his side. Candida became a health juggernaut.

CROOK'S VERSION OF CANDIDA

William Crook merged two separate concepts to create the candida hysteria: having too much candida and developing an allergy to it. These are really very different concepts, and they don't necessarily run together at all. You can have a dozen cats and not be allergic to any of them, or you can have no cats at all but wheeze and sneeze if you step for a moment into a house where one lived a year ago. But Crook melded "lots of cats" and "intense cat allergies," creating a nicely complex and weird diet that is just the ticket for orthorexic obsession.

The Candida diet has several main aspects. The first is a prohibition on eating sweets. Crook says that "sugar feeds yeast" and that therefore eating sweet foods increases the level of candida in your body. (He does not offer any meaningful proof for this statement; apparently our intestines are like wine bottles, and the more sugar you add, the faster the yeast goes to work.) This proscription includes fruit and fruit juice. An interesting unintended consequence of this part of the diet was that naturopathic dietary theories, previously in love with fruit, now began to shy away. This brought naturopathy closer to Chinese dietary beliefs, which relegate fruit to the role of an unhealthy dessert.

Of course, it is quite difficult to avoid all sweets, and unless you are unbelievably self-disciplined, you're guaranteed to slip up from time to time. Crook's writing encourages you to imagine a population explosion of candida in your body, accompanied by fatigue, headaches, sinus infections, and muscle pain. Believing makes it so, and therefore this feature of the diet is self-supporting.

Despite the lack of evidence for feeding yeast, refined sugar is certainly not a healthy food, and you can't go too wrong by minimizing it. Another aspect of the Candida diet is a bit more bizarre. It's a type of guilt by association. Crook forbids you to eat bread, because it contains bread yeast, tomato sauce because it contains mold, and even mushrooms because they all fall into the fungus family.

This recommendation is really rather far-fetched. While mushrooms, tomato mold, and bread yeast are indeed all fungi, they are not the fungus candida. The kingdom of fungi is large. You are no more likely to be allergic to mushrooms based on a candida allergy than to sneeze around elephants if you are allergic to mice. Crook is painting his allergies with a very broad brush when he sweeps all fungi together.

To make the dietary rule even odder, Crook sometimes appears to imply (and candida followers certainly believe) that eating mushrooms or tomato paste will increase the amount of candida in your body. This is extremely hard to understand, as one kind of fungus can't transform into another. To return to the previous analogy, acquiring mice will not fill your house with elephants.

Theoretically, one fungus *might* facilitate another's growth. However, this is unlikely, because fungi are generally enemies of one another, and in any case the fungi in bread and tomato paste at least are dead and can't do a lot of facilitating.

SYSTEMIC CANDIDIASIS?

As the candida theory took root in the culture, people began to generalize the idea, and some came to believe they had *Candida albicans* multiplying in their bloodstream. This led to the name "systemic candidiasis," a term that implies a body filled with yeast. The image is truly horrifying and has served to give added force to the fear driving candida. However, it's unreal. People with AIDS or advanced cancer may develop true systemic candidiasis (a potentially lethal complication), but practically no one else does. "Systemic candidiasis" as popularly used is a myth.

TREATMENTS FOR CANDIDA

The Candida diet fits well within the turf of natural medicine. So, too, does the use of *Lactobacillus acidophilus,* a friendly bacterium that fights candida. However, the candida hysteria soon left behind any reasonable definition of natural medicine and expanded into the realm of serious drugs. Crook himself recommended the drug nystatin, a safe but not very powerful medication. Interest then focused for a while on the WWII-era drug capryllic acid, now available over the counter. After a few years, however, people who believed they had candida no longer found these safe treatments effective. Supported by alternative practitioners, they turned to expensive and increasingly dangerous prescription pharmaceuticals, such as Sporonox, Diflucan, and the toxic medications ketoconazole and amphotericin B. Natural medicine used to be famous for saying "Treat the person and not the disease," but with candida the method is really identical to that of standard treatment: bring in the big guns and start shooting. In addition, a few natural products also made it onto the list of treatments, including grapefruit seed extract, garlic, oregano oil, and thyme oil.

This is all very much in the spirit of orthorexia. In the name of natural medicine, the obsession with one little fungus leads to the use of medications far from the realm of natural therapies. And does any of this really work? Not very well. Hundreds of my patients told me they had candida; they struggled endlessly with the diet, but practically none found anything like a cure for their symptoms. The benefit, if any, was almost always temporary.

Actually, this is only to be expected. There's no way to make candida go away permanently. It's a natural inhabitant of a healthy body. By means of various intensive regimens, you can make its numbers decrease, but only temporarily. The yeast will come back. It has to come back. And then, if you are truly allergic to it, you will feel sick again.

Fortunately, most people who believe they have a problem with candida really don't. The very idea of it is thankfully fading away. On the trendsetting West Coast, candida has gone the way of hypoglycemia; the newest trend involves intestinal amoebas said to cause cancer and pretty much all other diseases.

SIMPLE SOLUTIONS

Candida is an example of a simple solution: a unifying concept that is supposed to solve all life's problems. Raw-foodism is another, in its claim that cooked food is the source of all the world's problems. Similarly, macrobiotics attributes all world problems to an inadequate balance of yin and yang in the diet.

History is littered with many more beautiful simple solutions that didn't work out very well (think of Communism). Nonetheless, they remain perennially popular because they allow us to ignore the real complexity of life. What a relief!

Orthorexia is another simple solution. It frees us from thinking about the full range of issues that might matter in our lives and turns our attention toward one direction only: what goes into the mouth. It's wonderful! The only problem is that it's a lie.

If you have been following the Candida diet, loosen up. By all means avoid sweet foods if you feel better doing so, and if bread makes you sleepy, you can skip bread. But don't try to follow the diet perfectly, and above all, don't think that following it perfectly will solve all your health problems. Even at its best, diet isn't quite that powerful.

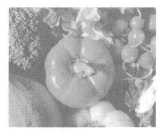

11.

Eat Right for Your Type?

While I think there's a lot of truth to the Zone diet and some truth to the Candida diet, while I respect the philosophy behind macrobiotics and the spiritual impulse behind raw-foodism, there is one up-and-coming diet I don't respect at all: the blood type diet. In my opinion it is ridiculously wrong.

I'm referring to the diet popularized in *Eat Right for Your Type* (Dr. Peter J. D'Adamo, Putnam, 1996). In case you haven't heard of it, this book provides highly specific dietary advice based on your blood type. The premise is that various blood types developed at certain points in evolutionary history, and therefore people with that blood type should eat what the people ate at that time. Type O evolved during the caveman period; therefore, individuals with that type should eat a great deal of meat; type A evolved toward the beginning of agriculture, so people with this blood type should eat a lot of grains. You get the picture.

This book has a certain appeal because it acknowledges one

definite fact: Different diets work well for different people. That's indubitably true, and the possibility of knowing which diet is best for you has caught the imagination of many, many people.

According to *Eat Right for Your Type*, type-O individuals should eat what amounts to a version of the Zone diet, type A's should eat a modified Mediterranean diet, type B and type AB get more peculiar dietary recommendations. Unfortunately, these recommendations are without foundation; or rather, the foundation offered doesn't support the house if you look at it closely.

We could start with the absurdity of assuming that a blood type embodies the genetics of an evolutionary period. Blood types are very tiny mutations; they are no more likely to capture the essence of, say, caveman life, than nose shape or eye color should.

Or we could look at how genetics works and point out that the time scales for adaptations to new diets simply aren't long enough for such sweeping genetic changes as the theory hypothesizes.

Or we could critique the amazing specificity of the book's suggestions and question how it could be known that bluefish is good but catfish is bad for type-O people.

And is it really responsible to say that type-A people really aren't allergic to peanuts, when peanut allergies are potentially fatal?

I wish there really were a scientific basis for deciding what kind of diet is best for you. If there were, I'd be recommending it enthusiastically. However, there isn't, not by a long shot. The apparent scientific foundation of this particular bestseller is an illusion.

We all trust science to a certain extent. When there isn't any science to guide us, we want to latch on to something. If information seems to come from an expert, and it sounds scientific, it can be very convincing. *Eat Right for Your Type* does contain some actual science, but then it so frequently loses track that's it's hard even to know where to start critiquing it. This is simply not a rational book. I could write a book called *Eat Right for Your Nose Type* with as much scientific foundation.

Of course, true believers, and the author, will violently attack my preceding comments. So I'll take another tack. Let's assume that the theory behind the book is correct and that your blood type really does determine what you should eat. By all means, go ahead and follow the suggestions. But please keep a sense of proportion.

Already in the last year I've met dozens of people using the blood type diet as a route to orthorexia. The immensely detailed dietary and lifestyle program it recommends is perfect fodder for obsession. You can spend most of your day trying to apply this book's principles, all the while comforting yourself with the notion that you are doing just the right thing. Never mind your personal preferences, desires, or intuitions. Just follow the book.

Imagine Maya, a twelve-year-old whose parents have adopted this approach. Mom is type A, Dad is type B, brother is type O, and Maya is AB. Each one is supposed to eat and live completely differently. The amount of time this family has to devote to following the principles of food will be enough to exhaust their creative energy for years.

And Maya hates the relaxation exercises the book tells her to practice. She wants to play soccer like her type-O brother. But only type O's should engage in aerobic exercise. She also wants to eat meat. But only her brother should eat meat. She's supposed to drink goat's milk. She hates goat's milk.

This diet is a way for her parents to control every aspect of her life. The best I can say is that in her case this book will provide a good future income to some nice psychotherapist who has to undo the damage.

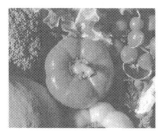

12.

Living on Tablets

Although orthorexia mostly involves extreme diets, it can occur in another form as well: a fixation on small, hard, round objects, piled high in the palm and swallowed with a tall glass of water. I am referring to vitamin pills and other food supplements. In my years of practicing alternative medicine, I met as many pill orthorexics as any other kind.

Nutritional supplements and herbal treatments certainly can offer health benefits. For example, there's no question that for many people it's a good idea to take extra calcium, and without doubt a multivitamin and -mineral tablet can serve as insurance against an inadequate diet. Furthermore, high-dose vitamin E supplements likely reduce the risk of heart disease and certain forms of cancer, and good scientific evidence tells us that many herbs are effective in the treatment of certain illnesses. In my other books and on the Web site I direct *(www.tnp.com)*, these rational uses of food supplements are thoroughly documented.

However, just as healthy eating can become obsessive, the use of vitamins and food supplements can get out of hand. When your natural pills start to multiply and you need a large shopping bag to carry them around, when the number of tablets you take daily is greater than the number of coins you typically find in your pocket, you've crossed the line and become an orthorexic pill user.

During my years of practice, patients frequently brought me pill-filled shopping bags accompanied by long lists of supplements. My ordinary response was to cross off enough to get the total number down to reasonable levels. Some patients have responded gratefully. But most have not. I have expended an enormous amount of energy over the years, with little result, trying to convince people that the stomach is not a bag to be filled up with pills. Frequently patients have become so angry at me that they've gotten up and walked out, offended by my heresy against the gods of tablets.

I've come to understand why conventional physicians so often prescribe antibiotics for colds, against their better judgment. It is simply very difficult to argue against the beliefs of a patient. And should one even argue? We know that the mind is a powerful thing in healing. If a person believes in pills, and they are safe pills, it is almost certain that the pills will help. Placebo tablets, after all, have been known to provide significant symptom relief in up to 90 percent of individuals who take them (the percentage varies with the disease). How much more effective should a complicated pill regimen be, with its innumerable opportunities for positive suggestion.

A colleague, whom I shall call Dr. J, has come to fully embrace the power of the placebo. A pill-worshipping patient named Karen convinced her. Here is the story in Dr. J's own words:

Karen was about thirty-two years old, active, energetic, the mother of three young children, and the proprietor of a home-based market research consultant business. She looked healthier than I, and when she asked me for advice on the precise hour of the day she should take her supplements, my mind took a critical turn.

"I ordinarily take my calcium aspartate at ten A.M. every day," Karen said thoughtfully, referring to her stack of yellow legal-size papers covered with script in red felt-tipped marker. "I'm thinking, however, that I should take it in the afternoon, perhaps three P.M., or even four P.M. And do you think I should substitute calcium gluconate for the aspartate a couple of days a week, so my system doesn't get too used to the one supplement?"

"Well . . ." I said, trying not to express my true feelings. Karen continued the conversation without any help from me.

"Another issue is my magnesium. I've heard that magnesium picolinate is ten percent better absorbed than magnesium aspartate, so I've been thinking that I should reduce my dose by ten percent. Of course, I take the magnesium at least two hours away from the calcium, to avoid absorption problems."

"Yes, very good," I said. I wanted to tell her that she was way too focused on supplements, but I didn't yet know her well enough to be confrontational.

"However, I don't know if I should take the magnesium at one in the afternoon, just after lunch, or hold off till two hours before dinner, so I can take the calcium with a meal."

I found myself thinking of a story I had just read in *The New Yorker*. As I recall it, a rather disreputable young man decides to make a change in his life and try something socially redeeming. The scheme he hits upon involves reading to a blind woman in her home.

He has never known a blind person before and takes immature delight in making strange faces at her while she talks. The fact that she can't see him, that all she hears is the unbroken stream of his reading, strikes him as hilarious and almost mystical.

I am amused to find myself doing the same thing. In my mind, where Karen can't see it, I hear myself saying, "Why don't you take one-fifth of a five-hundred-milligram pill of calcium aspartate at nine A.M., two-fifths of a three-hundred-milligram pill of calcium gluconate at ten A.M., and so on, alternating until three P.M., when you take one-tenth of a two-hundred-milligram pill of calcium citrate and one-twentieth of a six-hundred-milligram calcium carbonate tablet." But I don't say anything out loud.

She goes on, unaware of my internal dialogue. "I've been considering adding manganese to my regimen. What do you think of manganese? Chelated manganese, of course."

The *New Yorker* story continues in my brain, into the escalation scene where the protagonist begins silently drawing on the blind woman's walls in red crayon. A similar hysteria is building up in me, an impulse to go beyond my professional norms.

"Of course," Karen says, "you probably can give me all sorts of ideas I've never thought about. So I should stop talking and get your suggestions."

She carefully turns to a fresh yellow sheet and waits with her pen poised.

I try to formulate a sensible response. I really should tell her that she is trying too hard, that supplements don't deserve quite that much detailed attention. But I know from innumerable past patient encounters that she won't want to hear that from me. She desperately wants me to make up a story for her.

And I suddenly think that maybe I should. Karen loves supplements. Who am I to dissuade her? If she believes in them, they'll work.

Now that I've given myself permission, the fantasy in my brain bursts out through my lips. I launch into the most absurd pill-scheduling recommendation imaginable, while she hastily scribbles on the yellow legal pad. "Take calcium gluconate at ten A.M. and three P.M. on Tuesday and Thursday, at a dose of eighty-three milligrams (one-third of a two-hundred-fifty-milligram tablet). Then switch to a combination of calcium aspartate and calcium orotate on the other weekdays, taken both when you wake up in the morning (before eating) and just prior to dinner. However, on the weekend, I want you to dissolve a five-hundred-milligram tablet of calcium carbonate in orange juice three times daily. Not every weekend, though. On the second weekend of the month, leave out the calcium carbonate and instead take fifty milligrams of calcium lactate every two hours while awake, regardless of meals."

Karen is happily scribbling away.

I go on inventing an absurdly detailed schedule for fourteen other vitamins and minerals. It is perfectly correct in its total intake, but utterly imaginative in its specificity. Karen continues to nod happily and write it all down. Finally she has a set of instructions that cover seven legal pages. I declare the session over. Karen leaves, ecstatically pleased with me.

Two weeks later she calls me to report dramatic improvement in her symptoms. When I meet her on the street a month later, she introduces me to several of her friends as "the most knowledgeable nutritional physician she's ever known." I demur from that compliment but take note of the power of the placebo. Karen refers about thirty of her friends to me, all of whom come expecting similar regimens, and I provide them. Most of them do very well.

I understand why someone like Karen would want a fantasy regimen. I've been there myself. I know the extraordinary security that comes from a time-consuming self-care ritual. The day is cumbered about on all sides by brightly colored pills that say, "Everything will be all right." Simply trying to hold them all in mind drives out other anxieties, and the jolt of well-being each time they go down the throat is like a shot of pure vitality. The interior sensation is much like that created by a diet of raw, organically grown fruits and vegetables; a more digitalized assurance, but assurance nonetheless.

I don't know precisely how widely pill orthorexia is spread throughout the country, but it was quite common among my patients. For example, here is a yellow legal page I found sticking out of one of my medical charts from 1987 (altered for medical privacy reasons):

My Daily Schedule

8:00 A.M.   Take vitamin C, vitamin E, and calcium
8:25 A.M.   Take one tablespoon betaine hydrochloride; one ounce wheat grass concentrate
8:30–9:00 A.M.   Breakfast
9:00 A.M.   Take magnesium, zinc, manganese and copper supplements, with eight ounces of water
9:15 A.M.   Take liquid mineral supplement
9:30 A.M.   Time for Spirulina
10:00 A.M.   Take B-vitamin combination, plus extra vitamin B12 on Mon, Wed, and Fri. Six ounces of water
10:30 A.M.   Take ginkgo, grapeseed, and garlic capsules. Use aged garlic for one week, alternate with powdered garlic the next
11:30 A.M.   Take vitamin C, vitamin E, and calcium
11:55 A.M.   Take one tablespoon apple cider vinegar
12:00–12:30 P.M.   Lunch

You have to have a lot of time on your hands to follow a schedule like this.

THE ROMANCE OF PILLS

Part of the attraction of pills lies in the fact that they look like drugs. Even though they may contain natural substances, pills are clear or brightly colored objects that make a nice pile in the hand and go down the throat with a hefty swallow. For some of us it is easier to believe that a pill can fight disease and strengthen health than can a head of broccoli. Pills are active agents; they do something to you, carry out a mission in your body, seek out a goal that is more focused than the passive influence of a food.

Yet they are not drugs. Natural supplements also carry the cachet of herbs or health foods. When you put a drug in your mouth, it feels like a necessary evil at best. In contrast, a vitamin seems supercharged with nourishment; it's a shove in the right direction.

And you don't have to alter your eating habits or struggle against the tastes you've acquired over many years to adopt a pill regimen. Pills are easy, require no effort or sacrifice, and cost nothing but money and the ability to remember to take them. They are natural medicine without the bother of tofu, broccoli, and brown rice.

But do you ever imagine what all those pills look like in your stomach, rattling about like candy in a Halloween sack, slowly oozing away, releasing their concentrated chemicals against the lining of your digestive tract? It is ironic that vitamins, minerals, and other food supplements ever became part of the natural health movement. They are actually the opposite of natural foods. Food supplements, and even the currently popular herbal extracts, are refined, processed products. They resemble white sugar more than they do whole foods.

In the seventies and eighties there were two forms of stores catering to natural health: the health food store and the natural food store. The former focused on concentrates, the latter on food in its natural state: whole grains, fruits, and vegetables. Natural food stores avoided vitamin pills as a matter of principle. Influenced by the original theories of the natural foods movement, their crusade was against removing nutrients from the context in which nature made them. If even white flour with added vitamins (enriched flour) is the enemy, how much more inimical seems a pill containing nothing but vitamins and no real food at all?

To counter to this perception, health food stores offered "natural vitamins," an oxymoron like a "tame wolverine" or an "honest politician." A rose hip is a natural product that happens to be high in vitamin C, just as corn is a vegetable that is high in sugar. But vitamin C made from rose hips is no more natural than high-fructose corn syrup; actually, it is less natural, as it is more completely refined. Vitamins are not natural, even though they originated in a natural product. They are produced in chemical factories, just like prescription drugs that start their life in a plant constituent. The essence of the term "natural," as it is used all throughout alternative medicine, is that a substance remains close to its original form. Vitamins and minerals don't fit this formulation; they are part of the natural health movement by a historical accident, not because they belong there.

Linus Pauling was the main cause of this change. He so strongly championed vitamin C and aroused such hostility from the medical profession that alternative medicine felt inspired to take his side. From that point on, supplements became the mainstay of natural medicine, and ultimately even the natural food stores succumbed. Don't get me wrong. I'm not saying that vitamins and food supplements are bad. Far from it. I personally take several supplements: vitamin E to protect my heart, ginkgo extract to improve my memory, and calcium to keep my bones strong. And I, too, am reassured by placing these pills in my mouth. With little investment of time I can give myself a jolt of optimism about my health. I imagine them spreading out through my body bringing health and regeneration; in addition to their real benefits, I receive the benefits of positive self-suggestion.

Furthermore, the complicated pill regimens I described above have some basis in reality. There is absolutely no doubt that certain forms of supplements are absorbed better than others: calcium citrate than calcium carbonate, for example. Not only that, it is better to take some supplements on an empty stomach, others on a full stomach, while others are absorbed best if divided into relatively small doses and taken throughout the day.

But it can be pushed too far. As with all other forms of orthorexia, it's the obsession and not the facts that constitute the disease; there is a law of diminishing returns, where the benefits of supplements are outweighed by the fact of obsession.

How much of your day do you spend thinking about flossing your teeth? That's about the same amount of heart and mind you should devote to your supplements; it's a matter of good hygiene but not of self-fulfillment. But this is easily forgotten. Pills can come to embody a great symbolic power, actually taking on elements of religious infatuation.

MAGIC SUBSTANCE WORSHIP

I call this phenomenon "magic substance worship," and I include in it reverence for exotic herbs and the most newly minted miracle cure. Because I have succumbed to it myself, I have a definite sympathy for the impulse. However, this is perhaps the shallowest form of orthorexia, the one with the fewest redeeming features. There is no depth, no art, no holism, in it, just idolatry and materialism.

Drugs are not usually very romantic. Except for the cult of Dilantin (spearheaded by Jack Dreyfus of Dreyfus Mutual Funds, who believes that this anti-epilepsy medication has an enormous range of health benefits), I have seldom met a patient who idealized and extolled the virtues of a prescription drug. But magic substance worship plays a powerful and constant role in alternative medicine. I have met thousands of people with a full-blown mystical passion for the wonders of natural medicine, whether bee propolis, pycnogenol, barley magma, or a concentrated extract of *Vitex agnus-castus*.

Since the beginning of my professional involvement in the field, probably not one month has gone by without some marvelous new material demanding my attention, either through the words of a patient or by direct mail. Over the last couple of years some of the most popular have been MSM, pregnenolone, ozone, super blue-green algae (the successor to spirulina, itself now largely replaced in the public trust by barley magma), sheep thyroid, ciwujia, and kombucha tea, but a complete list would extend several pages.

Entire books have been written about any magic substance you can name. Some substances arrive justified by elaborate and highly speculative semiscientific arguments; others invoke the wisdom of the ascended masters and call for an act of faith.

The earliest magic substance I can recall is chlorophyll. Proffered as a cure-all soon after its discovery, chlorophyll was an important magic substance when I was a child. I remember a certain gum packed with chlorophyll that was sold at the counter of health food stores and later at the supermarket. It was supposed to cure headaches, allergies, ulcers, and colds. Chlorophyll has lost its charm today, but it gave rise to a succession of green magic substances, including wheat grass, spirulina, super blue-green algae, and barley magma. Each of these worked miracles for five or more years before it was pushed off its pedestal by something even greener and more bitter.

Some reverenced substances possess a long-standing pedigree. Goldenseal, for example, has been the subject of immense popular enthusiasm on and off since the early 1800s, when Samuel Thomson and his health cult raised it to the status of cure-all. The plants have been harvested to near-extinction many times and then forgotten for a decade or so, in a series of booms and busts resembling nothing so much as the business cycle. Today it is among the ten top-selling herbs, due to the false belief that it can disguise the results of a drug test or stimulate immunity. (Actually, goldenseal is mostly a topical antibiotic and perhaps also a type of decongestant.)

The Thomsonians also praised the herb lobelia as a marvel of healing, and its reputation so impressed Jethro Kloss that he gave it twenty-eight consecutive pages in *Back to Eden*. Traditionally you are supposed to take enough lobelia to make you vomit.

Ozone therapy, on the other hand, puts on the reputation of science to fashion its robes of glory. One suggested method of using it involves carrying substantial portions of your blood into tubes outside your body and then bubbling ozone through it. This is not exactly a natural therapy, although if you decide you want this treatment, you will have to find a practitioner of natural medicine. Ozone is certainly an interesting molecule, and its association with lightning gives it an aura of tremendous healing power. It's supposed to cure just about everything—cancer, heart disease, MS, even autism. (Please be advised: I don't recommend this unproven treatment.)

Certain personalities are attracted to certain cures. Ozone and hydrogen peroxide appeal to the technologically minded. Apple cider vinegar attracts those who trust folk wisdom. And kombucha tea tingles the imagination of those who believe that the East is the repository of secret healing wisdom.

If only healing were really as easy as swallowing a magic substance! But whether it's apple cider vinegar or royal jelly, it is unfortunately true that the testimonials drastically outweigh any real healing power. Magic substances have their time of glory, cure millions, and then lose all power when the spotlight shifts. It is the worship that makes the testimonials, not the healing power of the substance.

As with other forms of orthorexia, the danger in magic substance worship is not so much physical as psychological harm. Some treatments may actually be dangerous, but in most cases the problem is subtler. It is the materialism of substance worship that is the illness, the iconography of a green liquid, a brown powder, or a bad-tasting food. If we are going to worship something, let it be something that enlarges our horizons.

The nature of love is that it reshapes us into the image of what we love. If we love Mahatma Gandhi or Mother Teresa, our character expands, becomes grand and noble. If we love Adolf Hitler, we become the spitting image of his hatred and small-minded cruelty. If we love history, theater, mathematics, nature, or God, our soul also grows.

But what happens when we love a pill? Unlike a long walk by the river or a talk with a friend, pills narrow our life rather than expand it, shrink it to the size of a hard, round object rattling about in the palm of a hand. Food worship seems elevated by comparison. An orange, an apple, a loaf of bread—these at least have their own poetry. Pills are dead things, and when we worship them, we contract our lives.

WHY PILLS SEEM TO WORK

But, you may argue, you know someone cured by one of the supplements I've just finished maligning. How can I claim them to be so worthless?

I will readily admit that these revered materials occasionally do cure. Not usually, but sometimes. This used to confuse me terribly. I used to assume that if a treatment could cure once, it must be a pretty powerful treatment. It took me a long time to understand otherwise. The case of Pearl O'Shaughnessy comes to mind as a good example.

I first met Pearl one year prior to the prolonged illness that I'll soon describe. She came striding into my office talking quickly and loudly: about Chinese kickboxing, marathon horseback riding, and the "flimsiness" of every man she had ever known.

By profession, Pearl was, surprisingly, a podiatrist; her personality suggested a mixture of Alexander the Great and Katharine Hepburn. She stood about five foot eleven, wore cowboy boots, and dressed all in black.

"I don't think you can help me, you know," she began. "But tell me this. Why do I wake with a thumping headache every morning?"

After questioning her, I suggested that it might be related to the chocolate candy she ate every night before going to bed. We discussed hypoglycemia at length. I gave her several practical suggestions that I thought might help. After she left that first visit, I recall reflecting that this was a patient who was far healthier than I.

I did not hear from the powerful podiatrist for nearly a year. When she arrived at my office the following autumn, she seemed an altogether different woman.

Speaking quietly and indistinctly, Pearl explained that following a flu in early spring, she had never recovered her energy. For all of the last six months she had not been able to work for more than two hours at a stretch without feeling as if she wanted to collapse. This crippling exhaustion was ruining her career and the rest of her life.

"I feel lazy, weak, content to sit on the couch," she admitted shamefacedly. "*Sit on the couch*—that's something I never used to do. I can't even get up on a horse's back. Going out to the movies seems like a lot these days."

The medical workup for unexplained fatigue is endless. We performed an immense battery of diagnostic tests, without finding a single clue. Her thyroid gland continued to pump out sufficient thyroid hormone; her liver revealed no signs of chronic hepatitis; her blood count demonstrated no anemia or signs of infection; she did not show any evidence of internal inflammation or any autoimmune processes. So far as the gleaming machines of the lab were concerned, Pearl was healthy.

But she was not healthy. This was not Pearl O'Shaughnessy; this was a shadow of the kickboxing podiatrist. I toyed briefly with the idea that she might have Chronic Fatigue syndrome. However, Pearl did not exhibit any of the other signs, such as chronic sore throat and lymph gland swelling.

After about six weeks of testing and referral to specialists, I gave up hope I would ever find a medical cause. This did not discourage me, however. Many illnesses cannot be fully diagnosed, perhaps even the majority, if the truth be told. I could still treat her with alternative medicine.

I tried all the techniques I knew to cure unexplained fatigue. I performed acupuncture, prescribed herbs, experimented with various supplements, and sent her to be Rolfed. In my experience one of these methods will almost always work for fatigue. But in Pearl's case it was all to no avail. She was still exhausted, still not a tenth of the person she used to be.

So I decided to look for body/mind causes. I wondered whether Pearl's body was informing her that she needed to become more balanced. She had been all activity with no time for quiet, all action and no repose. Perhaps that was the meaning of the fatigue—perhaps it was a forceful invitation from Pearl's deepest self. Perhaps she was being called upon to balance her ferocious lifestyle by practicing the arts of stillness.

I thought I was brilliant when I suggested this possibility to her. However, Pearl did not appreciate my eloquence. "I don't want to meditate," she said. "I don't want to gaze at scenery, to write in a journal, or go on spiritual retreats. I want to ride my horse for thirty miles at dawn. I want to compete in rodeos. I want to get married again; that is, if I can find a man who's man enough to match me!"

I admired her defiance, but it did not sound realistic anymore. Her pasty complexion and the obvious heaviness in her limbs and spirit seemed to make her ambitions ludicrous. She had been diminishing for eight months or more. She looked so sick that, if I had not met the marvelous Pearl O'Shaughnessy of the year before, I would have thought this person before me had always suffered from poor health.

We went around and around for many sessions. I tried to interest her in the beauty of a balanced life, to make the quest for moderation as exciting and difficult as winning a blue ribbon for lassoing steers. I spoke of the need to find healing from within, painstakingly explaining that not all medicine comes from the outside. Despite my best efforts, Pearl remained unconvinced. She did not get better, and eventually she stopped coming to see me.

Several months later I called Pearl at her podiatry clinic to see how she was doing. I hoped she might be ready to come around to my way of looking at things.

"Oh, yes, Dr. Bratman, how good of you to call. I'm all better now." Her voice sounded surprisingly bright and energetic.

I was taken aback. "What? You are? Er, well, now, that's wonderful. How did you do it?"

"It was easy. I went to see this man named Dr. L. He solved the problem for me right away."

I fumed to hear that name. Dr. L is a notorious "hit-and-run healer." With his mail-order Ph.D. in nutrition, he travels from state to state, selling whichever products currently appeal to him. I had known about him for years. I ate dinner with him once. In my opinion he is a classic flake.

I sputtered but tried to maintain my dignity. "That's wonderful to hear, Pearl. I am . . . um, so glad you found what you needed. Would you mind telling me what he gave you that helped so much?"

"Not at all. It's a miracle cure! Everyone should know about it. It's his own highly purified form of a recently discovered enzyme called CoQ10."

I chewed on my knuckles. Recently discovered? Bosh! Highly purified? Yeah, right. Try steaming the label off, Pearl. It's just repackaged health food store CoQ10, if I know my Dr. L.

"It's marvelous stuff, absolutely incredible," she gushed. "It prolongs life, makes you live past a hundred; prevents senility, enhances energy, and clears the mind. It gave me back all my strength and more, in a couple of weeks. I'm back on the rodeo circuit! If I stop it, though, I start to fade. So I plan to take it forever." Her voice thrilled with energy. "CoQ10 is concentrated cool power. It was just what I needed."

All at once her tone changed. Pearl seemed to notice my position suddenly, to realize that I might consider myself a failure. Charitably, she offered me a chance to save face. "You know, Dr. B, you were right what you said to me back then. I did need more balance. Only it wasn't meditation I needed. It was CoQ10. That stuff has given me balance. Its energy is calm and even, not at all like my past wildness. So you did help me, Dr. B. I thank you for that."

Humph! That was not what I meant at all! I had been talking about inner healing, not about taking a *pill!* However, I kept quiet. I was polite. But Pearl wasn't done with me.

"By the way, Dr. Bratman, I'm selling CoQ10 myself now. You could use a little more energy yourself, a little more oomph. Maybe you should buy some."

Stuttering, feeling about as adequate as Elmer Fudd, I congratulated her on her good fortune, thanked her for her offer, and hung up. I happened to know where to find Dr. L then, so I called him.

"Excellent job you did with Pearl O'Shaughnessy, Dr. L," I oozed in as sincere a voice as I could manage.

"Oh, yes, Pearl. A delightful woman. I've enjoyed working with her very much."

"I'm very glad to hear that," I replied, trying not to huff. "I wonder if you could tell me, how did you know to give her CoQ10? It was obviously a brilliant insight into the case."

Mumbling slightly, he explained, "Well, yes, actually, I give it to all my patients with fatigue. It cures them every time. You see," he began pedantically, "CoQ10 is a substance that occurs naturally in the mitochondria. The mitochondria are portions of nearly every cell that have the job of extracting energy from glucose and other molecules."

"Yes, yes, I know that," I interrupted with some heat. I knew what some promoters of CoQ10 claim. They say that since the mitochondria help produce bodily energy, and since CoQ10 is an essential part of the mitochondria, it follows that supplementing the diet with CoQ10 will increase energy.

This is a very weak chain of reasoning. One might as well argue that since spark plugs help produce energy inside the motors of cars, ground-up spark plugs should be added to the gas tanks of sluggish vehicles. The logic is absurd. It is classic pseudoscience.

But CoQ10 had cured Pearl O'Shaughnessy after nearly a year of illness. I could hardly deny the fact. It couldn't have been a spontaneous remission, for the symptoms returned whenever she stopped taking the supplement.

I hate cures like this. Sloppy thinking shouldn't lead to methods that work. But it sometimes happens.

"I understand the . . . um, reasoning behind CoQ10, Dr. L," I continued. "What I wonder is this: How often does it work when you prescribe it?"

"I find it very often useful and efficacious" he replied after a pause.

"Can you give me a rough estimate of what percentage of the time it helps?" I pressed.

"Well, not a percentage, really. But CoQ10's effects on cellular metabolism are very convincing. The mitochondria are the powerhouses of the cells, you know, and—"

I interrupted with scant courtesy, "Yes, *yes,* I know the speculative explanation. What I want to know is how often does it actually succeed?"

He did not know.

In my experience every remedy, without exception, succeeds occasionally. I did not realize this twenty years ago, when I began to study alternative medicine. I used to believe that if one person rids himself of rheumatoid arthritis with, say, propolis, the same method should work for nearly everyone who repeats the experiment. Certainly there might be an occasional failure. But if a substance can cure— really cure, dramatically, even once—it must be powerful medicine!

As my experience grew, I discovered the wide prevalence of failure. Supplements and herbs that work marvelously for one individual fail miserably for a dozen others. Testimonials do not generalize. For example, low doses of oral vitamin B12 produced one incontrovertible cure of severe childhood asthma in 1949, in a famous case quoted widely by nutritionists. Does this mean that oral vitamin B12 is a great treatment for asthma? No! It hardly ever works.

The list of impressive and dramatic cures is endless. Every book on alternative medicine is full of miraculous case histories. I believe that many of these stories are true. But magic substances, it seems, dislike encore performances. A particular remedy may work for no more than one in a thousand patients. Why not simply start at one end of a health food store and gradually work through to the other? That is probably nearly as useful as visiting someone like Dr. L.

But by some mysterious process, Pearl was cured. Inwardly I began to imagine that CoQ10 was a kind of concentrated, pearly energy. In my mind's eye it glowed with a pure, calm, and balanced strength, representing the titanic power of Pearl O'Shaughnessy sublimated into a capsule. It was with this impression in mind that I tried CoQ10 on sixteen fatigued patients in the subsequent months.

It failed every time. But I wouldn't give up. If Dr. L could do it, so could I! Two years after Pearl, CoQ10 cured one of my patients with dramatic suddenness. A very long history of chronic fatigue evaporated in two weeks, and she remained strong and energetic (though not so much as Pearl O'Shaughnessy) over the next several years that I knew her.

That patient still raves about me. "He knew just what to give me," she says. I am too craven to disillusion her. I actually have no idea why magic substances sometimes live up to their name but mostly slouch along taking your worship and your money without giving you anything in return.

Sometimes it is undoubtedly just the placebo effect; in other cases there may be some relatively rare and unrecognized condition in which a certain magic substance supplies precisely the missing ingredient to make the body work well again.

But how do you know? Taking up the most recent enthusiasm of a friend is very unlikely to help you. Recommendations from relatives may be more meaningful, because it is at least conceivable that you share a common genetic defect that can be fixed by a certain miracle nutrient. But most of the time, the overwhelming majority of the time, a new magic substance will help you only as long as your enthusiasm for it lasts; depending on how suggestible you are, its benefits will wear off in a week to two months. Soon you will find yourself taking up a new supplement. Your good friends will nod knowingly and put up with you as you switch supplement religions overnight and start a new evangelical campaign.

There's nothing wrong with trying supplements one after the other. A trial-and-error search for a substance that might help you, among options that are all generally rather safe, is an expensive but perfectly reasonable choice.

Still, perhaps it would be easier on those who love you if you would wait for a year before jumping on the recommendation bandwagon, a time period that might allow you to know whether or not it really works. And if you start turning to shopping bags to hold your purchases, if your supplement regimen begins to approach the complexity of a religious practice, when your friends begin to complain that *all* you ever talk about is pills, it may be worthwhile then to take a look at yourself and decide whether you are using your time and energy in the best possible way. Do you really want to make your life orbit around small, hard, round objects?

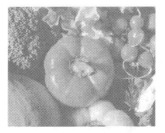

13.

The Beer and
Pizza Diet

The dietary approach described in this chapter can boast at least *two* testimonials. Unfortunately, this is not enough on which to base a bestselling diet book, or my fortune would be made. However, the fact that it was so successful in the following two cases made a deep impression on me and has helped me to remember that there's a lot more to health than food.

When she first came to see me, Lisa already lived a rather healthy lifestyle. She was a third-year chiropractic student who religiously followed a semivegetarian diet, exercised regularly, and drank a lot of water. The only real flaw in her lifestyle was a certain lack of sleep, such as might be expected of someone in chiropractic school. Still, overall, her self-care was distinctly above average. It struck her as unfair, therefore, when she began to develop a new bladder infection every couple of weeks, despite her daily consumption of a quart of cranberry juice. In fact, it was driving her crazy. Each infection required treatment with antibiotics, which gave her a yeast infection that itself needed treatment. She was ready and motivated for alternative medicine to help her, and I was sure I could help.

I tried everything I knew, methods that had worked well with so many others, such as herbs, supplements, acupuncture, and yoga postures. However, the infections still came back like clockwork. After a while I developed a theory that food allergies might be irritating her bladder and making her more susceptible to infection. Sure enough, food allergy testing came back with a list of significant allergies, and although I don't really trust the results of those tests, we decided to try eliminating all the proposed offenders. There were a lot of offenders, and the ultimate diet she wound up eating was pretty strict.

Nonetheless, being highly motivated, she followed it diligently for months. At the end of each month she came back to me with another bladder infection. It was terribly frustrating, because I had really expected to be able to help her. Usually, chronic bladder infections aren't that hard to treat. I was terribly tempted to take revenge on her for refusing to get well by accusing her of "cheating" on her diet.

I'm glad I held my tongue. For she eventually cured herself by means of an approach that was so unorthodox any criticism on my part would have made me, in hindsight, look like an even bigger fool.

After seeing me for a year, Lisa disappeared from my practice for six months. The following spring I saw her name on my day's list of appointments and looked forward to finding out what methods she had tried in the meantime. I have always learned a lot from my patients, and if she had discovered a new technique, I wanted to know what it was.

Her appearance was promising. The exhausted, bags-under-the-eyes look had vanished. She was radiant, energetic, and cheerful.

"No bladder infections for five months now," she said, without further introduction.

"How'd you do it?" I asked, suddenly feeling afraid that she had found a healer who was better than me.

"By diet."

"Ah," I said. I must have missed some foods she was allergic to. "What did you cut out?"

"Nothing," she said. "I put back in."

I raised my eyebrows. She hesitated.

"Actually," she said, after a pause, "I put myself on a beer and pizza diet."

She looked me in the eye. She was a chiropractic student; she believed in healthy food as much as I. We shared a moment of astonishment together and then burst out laughing. She explained that her new healing diet consisted of eating pizza and drinking beer at least four days a week and paying practically no attention to diet the rest of the week.

Overall, the way she ate wasn't really too bad; she avoided sugar and voluntarily consumed a great many fruits and vegetables. But pizza? Beer? Why should those foods help?

I speculated that it might be the lycopene in the tomatoes or the B vitamins in the beer?

She had her own theory. "What I needed to do was relax," she said. "Loosening up on food is what cured me."

The same diet also cured Paul. He came to me seeking help for the severe autoimmune disease lupus. His joints ached, he felt sick as if with a flu, and his kidneys were already showing signs of the damage that is lupus's most life-threatening effect.

I interviewed him extensively and made my recommendations. I had him become a vegetarian, take supplements, and start yoga. I also talked him into seeing a therapist. I thought he had some inner rage that was making his body attack itself. It seemed to me that by releasing his anger into punching bags and pillows, he would end up taking some of the pressure off his illness.

I worked with him for a number of months and felt rather satisfied with the good work I was doing. I had really remade his life for him.

However, after about six months, he had a lupus flare-up, felt much worse, got disgusted, and blew up at me. "You've got me eating like some sort of monk, and I'm no better! I beat pillows, cry, shout, stand on my head, but I'm dying. It isn't fair!"

"Well," I replied mildly, "it isn't so bad, such a tragedy that you have a healthy lifestyle, is it? Even if it hasn't helped your lupus, it is still good. You haven't lost anything by it."

Paul paused to ponder my wise comment, but perhaps he was just counting to ten hoping to avoid punching me. When he started talking, his tone was scathing. "You may believe that spending your whole life thinking about health is a good thing, but I don't. I think it's a damn waste of time. If I were to die tomorrow, I would consider that these last six months went down the drain. I'm not putting up with it a minute more!"

"But everyone thinks these things are good for you: healthy food, exercise, expression of feelings . . ." I said soothingly.

Paul stood up. "Obviously you do—and you should. You make your living that way."

"And," I continued, "how do you know it didn't help? Maybe otherwise you'd be worse."

He stormed out, unconvinced by my brilliant (and self-serving) argument. It was eight months before I saw him again. When I read his name on my appointment book, I expected a repentant fellow. But I was wrong. He was triumphant. His lupus had gone into full remission.

"How did you do it?" I asked, upset at having been proven so wrong.

"By putting myself on the same beer and pizza diet that worked for your patient Lisa. I met her at a party, and she showed me the path of true healing."

Based on these two experiences, perhaps I really should start a new dietary theory, the beer and pizza theory. Maybe the body's attempt to metabolize the alcohol, in the presence of all the B vitamins from the beer, causes it to process the essential fatty acids found in the olive oil of the pizza in such as way as to— It's always easy to come up with some clever-sounding explanation.

I could make a fortune on it, I guess. But I'd rather take another message home: that health is very complicated, and that sometimes relaxing and enjoying yourself is more important than being so very careful.

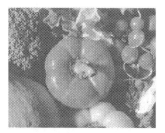

14.

How Well Do
Extreme Diets Work?

As we have seen, there are many different types of diets, which all contradict each other while at the same time all asserting that each is the one true way to eat. Each has its testimonials and its religious converts; each can take up an inordinate amount of space in your interior life.

Of course, if a diet or a magic substance were to produce a tremendous improvement in your health, it might be worth the sacrifice of a bit of obsession. Even so, you would eventually want to quit thinking about the method and just use its results to go on to live a life with your newfound health.

But how often do these diets really heal? Do they work as well as the stories say? And if they are so brilliant, why do they all contradict one another?

The contradictions certainly are amazing. For example, in her book *The Hippocrates Diet*, Ann Wigmore sketches out one of the classic versions of the raw foods diet. To bolster her claims for the efficacy of dietary treatments, she refers to the traditions of Chinese medicine. "They used natural therapies to heal for 5,000 years," she says. That's quite true. However, Wigmore fails to mention that any practitioner of Chinese medicine would enthusiastically condemn the Hippocrates diet as fundamentally mixed up and guaranteed to cause innumerable illnesses. Oriental medicine simply doesn't go well with raw foods theory.

Later in the same book Wigmore claims that a high-protein diet causes cancer. What would Zone dieters say?

The contradictions are endless. With all these competing theories and systems, it is hard for someone who is not an adherent of a particular system to believe that Ann Wigmore, or ancient Chinese doctors, or Barry Sears, or any other dietary expert has discovered the true way to eat.

Besides all the contradictions, there is a more fundamental question: Do any of these healing diets work?

HITTING THE JACKPOT

If you talk to a proponent of a dietary theory, you will of course hear nothing but stories of miracle cures. But if you ask a practitioner who is not sold on any particular method and keeps an open mind toward all of them, you will get a very different answer. In real life, extreme diets work about as often as the CoQ10 cure described previously, which is to say, not very often.

Then where do the testimonials come from? The truth is that even treatments with a low success rate can easily produce a raft of testimonials. For example, suppose there were a new drug for neck pain that failed 97 percent of the time but produced dramatic benefits in 3 percent of those who used it. By most standards this is a lousy treatment. It practically never works; the FDA would never approve it.

But then suppose that a hundred thousand people use the drug. Careful interviews of those participants would supply three thousand glowing testimonials! All you'd have to do is fail to report the disgruntled majority, and you could make an impressive case for the power of this usually worthless drug.

The same goes for extreme healing diets. Most people who try them don't get much in the way of obvious benefit. Many people actually feel worse, developing stomach upset, fatigue, or strange symptoms. But just as Coenzyme Q10 sometimes produces outstanding results, any diet you can name occasionally makes contact with something deep inside the body and causes dramatic improvements in quality of life.

In my years of practice as an alternative physician, I have certainly seen people cure themselves of serious diseases by means of dietary changes. The results I've seen with food allergy treatment are among the most impressive, with occasional apparent cures of autoimmune diseases such as lupus and rheumatoid arthritis, chronic hepatitis, asthma, depression, and dozens of other illnesses. Without formal statistics I have no idea what the percentage of cure really is. My overall impression from the stories I've heard is that food allergen identification and avoidance seldom helps more than a little, but occasionally it hits the jackpot.

Besides food allergies, I have met people benefited by almost every other diet you could name. One strange week I met two people with MS, one who had failed to improve on a raw foods diet while showing a miraculous recovery with macrobiotics, the other the reverse! It's all very strange and unpredictable; clearly there's more here than meets the eye.

AN OPTIMISTIC THEORY ON
WHY DIETS MIGHT WORK

I have an optimistic (although completely hypothetical) theory that might explain why widely varying diets seem to work for different people. The argument starts as follows: Animals clearly have a built-in system of knowing what they have to eat to get the nutrients they need. Otherwise, they wouldn't get all their essential nutrients, and they would die of malnutrition. Just as we feel thirsty when we lack water and know about how much to drink to supply the deficit, animals must also feel a craving for plants or mineral deposits when they need certain nutrients and seek them out.

It is not necessary to assume that animals instinctively know what foods will work. Perhaps they try different things, and their bodies then register what nutrients are provided. This would give them more flexibility to adapt to new environments.

Presumably people have the same ability, although, as with many of our innate abilities, living a complex, civilized life may have buried it to some extent.

Now, here's the next step in my reasoning: Perhaps the same system that allows animals to know what foods to eat allows them to eat differently when they are sick. Foods contain thousands of chemicals besides basic nutrient; perhaps our bodies are designed to be able to utilize those chemicals in order to correct certain health problems.

According to this theory, one person might need a certain odd diet while another person needs a completely different one, depending on the exact nature of the circumstances or the type of illness. Furthermore, a diet that helps me one year might not be what I need the next year. This is pure speculation, of course, but it could be the explanation for the impressive effects of such impressively inconsistent approaches.

WHICH DIET SHOULD YOU PICK?

But even if this theory is true, it isn't very helpful. How are you supposed to know what you should eat? When civilized people try to check their instincts about what to eat, too often the gauge reads "chocolate." We have moved so far from an instinctive animal existence that very few of us can properly "hear" what our body is saying.

Some alternative practitioners use a method called "applied kinesiology" to identify what foods or supplements would be right for their clients. On the face of it, the technique seems rather silly. You hold a certain food in your hand (or even just think about it) while the practitioner tests the strength of your arm muscles. Supposedly, weakness in muscle strength indicates that the food is bad for you, and increased strength suggests that it is healthful.

There are numerous more complex versions of this method, with fancy names like contact reflex analysis, and practitioners attend impressive seminars that last all weekend to become certified in this method. The best I can say about it is that it might be a way of contacting your hidden instincts regarding what to eat.

However, in real life, practitioners seem to always come up with recommendations that fit their personal dietary beliefs. Furthermore, if two different practitioners test the same person, the results don't agree.

If only there were some wise healer one could consult who knew exactly which diet would work best for us! I'd love to be able to ask whether I should go on Edgar Cayce's Jonathan apple fast, eat nothing but orange-colored food for a year, or adopt the beer and pizza approach. I have reason to believe that just the right diet might solve my health problems, but I don't know which one it is.

If someone really knew the answer, what a service it would be! Unfortunately, healers who claim to know usually just have an agenda to push. When I've spent time talking with them, I've realized they have no special knowledge. What they have is the chutzpah to tell people what to do based on no real understanding at all. Honest healers usually admit that it's all trial and error for them.

The blood type diet claims to know the secret key to the ideal way to eat, but I would put it in the chutzpah category. It gives solid and individualized advice; however, the basis of that advice is, to me, more than highly suspect. It is ludicrous.

Ayurvedic medicine, the traditional medicine of India, also offers individualized dietary plans. They are based on the categories Vatta, Pitta, and Kapha. Vatta people are thin, introspective, and easily fatigued; Kapha people are heavy, calm, and patient; and those in the Pitta category are high-energy, fast-moving, quick-to-anger types. The diet for each of these types is quite different from that for the others, and by combining a few types you can come up with a total of at least six diets. However, none of them agree with the blood type diet or any other system; they seem to help sometimes, and sometimes not.

Classic Chinese medicine has its own approach that comes up with dozens of diets based on "energetic patterns." Again, while these seem to be helpful for some, for others they simply don't "touch" the illness at all.

Are there hundreds or thousands of ways of eating, each with its own influence on health and appropriate to a given person in a given situation, and the only problem is that it is simply hard to find the right one? Or is there a less idealistic explanation?

A LESS PLEASANT THEORY

There is another possible explanation for the occasional healing miracles caused by diet besides the one I presented earlier. Let me warn you, if you are a fan of alternative healing, you are not going to like this theory.

It is quite possible that the healing benefits of some extreme diets may be entirely or at least greatly due to the power of suggestion. Perhaps the trappings, effort, and atmospherics behind various diets act as a kind of placebo, working the occasional healing miracles we read about.

People who feel that they have been healed by a diet will not wish to believe that this could be so. For some reason it is extremely annoying to think that one has been healed through the power of the mind. It is just fine for other people to be healed that way, but no one wants to think that all the trouble he or she went through to follow an arduous diet ended up simply creating an atmosphere of positive suggestion. Furthermore, it seems impossible that a dramatic cure could be caused by the power of the mind alone.

Still, if you look at it honestly, the possibility starts to look quite likely. The mind is very powerful. If it can cure cancer, it can cure other illnesses, too. There is very little doubt that, among its other effects, a complex dietary theory acts as a form of positive visualization. Every time you put a certified "healthy" food into your mouth, you imagine powerful health effects flooding your body; when you go through the sacrifice of avoiding Häagen-Dazs ice cream, an interior sensation of "I deserve good health for this" floods the mind.

This is all positive visualization. Is it any different in principle from imagining little cops zooming through your body zapping cancer cells? Whatever else they do, healing diets should focus the mind on healing and renew that focus many times a day.

One obvious objection to this theory is that you might have tried one diet to no effect and then found a cure with another. If it were merely the power of suggestion, shouldn't the first diet have worked? Not necessarily. The complex philosophical notions that underlie many dietary theories are part of the positive suggestion. A particularly meaningful theory might unlock your mind, so to speak. For example, macrobiotics tells you that through eating a proper mixture of yin and yang foods you will attune yourself to the universe. What a positive thought! Or, "When I eat raw foods, I fill myself with the raw energy of life." The more meaningful the dietary philosophy you follow, the greater the influence on the heart and mind, and the more significant one would expect the positive suggestion to be. If the philosophy happens to resonate well with the makeup of your personality, the structure of your deep needs, the effect will be even greater.

Dietary philosophies may also have positive psychological effects that improve your overall well-being. This in turn should increase your ability to heal. For example, if you are a person obsessed with control, macrobiotic theory gives you full scope for this control and, paradoxically, may help you relax in other aspects of your life. Raw-foodism may take a stultified, "couch potato" sort of person and put him in touch with a healthy primitive wildness. The obsessive avoidance suggested by food allergy methods may satisfy a need to say no to parts of life, thereby catalyzing a healing emotional release. The ultimate effect may be a surprisingly powerful influence toward healing, due not to the diet itself but to its many effects on the mind, heart, and spirit.

When scientists study drugs, herbs, or supplements, they use double-blind, placebo-controlled studies to factor out the power of suggestion. One group is given a real treatment, the other a placebo, and neither the study participants nor the researchers know who's who (until the study ends). Both groups usually get better, but the difference between the two groups shows how much is due to the treatment itself, beyond the placebo effect.

However, you can't do this with diets. Can you imagine not knowing if you were eating raw foods? This limitation on possible research makes it very difficult to know for sure how much of an outcome is due to a diet itself.

SYNERGY OF MIND AND DIET

Perhaps a more palatable theory combines two forces: the power of the mind and the content of the food.

Suppose that a diet does produce a physical effect through its biochemical content. This will work synergistically with the power of the mind as follows: Benefits due to the foods themselves will encourage the mind to trust the diet, thereby increasing the strength of the automatic positive visualization that goes along with choosing foods. In turn, suggestive effects will amplify the potency of the direct physical benefits. This is a powerful spiral that under the right circumstances might produce surprisingly powerful effects.

This is how I understand Louise's story. The two influences in her case were, on the biochemical level, the herb feverfew, and on the psychological level, her faith in me.

Faith in the authority who prescribes a diet or a treatment is a powerful factor in all healing through the power of the mind. Sometimes the charismatic founder of a major school of diet provides a great deal of that diet's power. For example, Michio Kushi, the popularizer of macrobiotics, seems to carry so much wisdom and understanding that just to hear him talk is to feel better. He presents his theory of macrobiotics with so much confidence and sublime wisdom that its truth seems unquestionable.

In a sense this is a form of faith healing: faith in a person or, more precisely, in the dream behind the person. We invest power in anyone who fits the mold of our dreams, and we tend to see the dream and not the person. We see a guru behind a long gray beard, detect a perfect mate on the evidence of a single smile, and imagine we have discovered a great healer after hearing a single anecdote or lecture.

I, too, have wanted so much to find a healer who is wise, caring, and potent that I've pretended to have found him—even though the person to whom I was speaking was only a full-size cardboard cutout of the healer of my dreams. I've made this error many times in my own searches for healing. The supposed mantle of greatness has also been dumped on my shoulders as a practitioner, with results that have astounded me.

Louise placed this kind of faith in me, and through it cured herself of a long-standing and serious health problem. She used an herb rather than a diet, but otherwise the process was similar. Her healing probably had something to do with the herb itself, and even more with the power of the mind. The episode I describe here shook me deeply.

Louise looked about sixty years old when I first saw her, but her chart said she was forty. Her off-balance posture spoke of chronic discomfort. As I studied her, I noticed that the muscles around her left eye were in a state of contraction, giving her face a lopsided appearance.

"Does the left side of your head hurt?" I asked her.

Louise gave me a look of astonishment. "How did you know that? I never told you that. I never told him that, did I?" She lifted up her palms, as if addressing God.

Though tempted to play the part of a magical clairvoyant healer, I confessed the prosaic source of my information.

"Well, you couldn't be more right," she continued, with amazement undiminished by the explanation. "I have these head explosions that tear the top of my skull right off. They last for three days at a time. I can't do anything with myself while they go on."

I tried screwing up my face in the same fashion as Louise. Imitating her expression made me hurt from my forehead down to my left shoulder. I asked her if her neck hurt. Direct hit! She said her entire left neck and shoulder throbbed and burned, even on a good day.

This rather simpleminded inference gave me her complete confidence. In the story that made the rounds later, it was said that I figured out all of Louise's problems without her telling me a single thing. "Dr. Bratman can just look at you and know everything that's wrong with you," she told her friends. "He must be psychic."

Unfortunately, I'm not psychic. Most of the time I don't know anything. To alleviate my ignorance, I asked Louise a thousand questions. She enjoyed the attention and particularly appreciated it when I asked, "Now, tell me, Louise, do you have any other symptom I have not asked about? It doesn't have to be a real problem, just something unusual, anything that doesn't feel quite right."

Louise responded with a long list of interesting sensations and quirky feelings. She was clearly grateful that I had asked, as I knew she would be. Everyone complains that conventional physicians don't seem interested in finding out much about their patients. "He didn't want to hear a word I had to say," Louise said about a previous doctor. "You're completely different."

Actually, the reason most doctors don't ask many questions is that there is not a lot they can do with the information. There are only so many key symptoms; regarding headaches, once you've asked the questions that differentiate among the various types of headaches and possible underlying causes, there isn't really much else to inquire about.

However, at that time I practiced acupuncture and Chinese medicine. This approach to healing has its own set of important symptoms to identify. Because Americans are not as familiar with them as they are with the verbal tool kit of conventional medicine, these points of consideration appear original and open-ended. Actually, I was listening for some very specific key words, too, and when I heard them, I made notes. Everything else flew by me.

Among those that I could connect successfully within the framework of Chinese medicine include heat in the palms, feet, and chest; inner restlessness; dry mouth; bladder urgency (without a bladder infection); cracked nails; scanty menstrual periods; insomnia; an occasional tremor; limbs frequently falling asleep; and muscle spasms in the legs. Just like "squeezing chest pain radiating to the neck and left arm, sweating and shortness of breath" immediately catches the attention of any physician, when juxtaposed these aforementioned health items form a classic menagerie of symptoms any first-year acupuncture student could identify.

Louise also reported a collection of signs and symptoms I could not integrate at all, including small blisters on the chin, a sensation of throbbing in both ring fingers, two episodes of gallbladder pain without gallbladder disease, frequently stubbed toes, and hair loss on the left side of the scalp only. I agreed with Louise that these miscellaneous symptoms no doubt contained some information about her body, but I did not know what to make of them, and although I wrote them down, I immediately forgot about them.

Nonetheless, in the rendition Louise spread around town, I was "the first doctor who could put every one of my symptoms together with the other ones to make a complete picture."

I then moved to a series of psychological questions. Not surprisingly, these quickly revealed a history of childhood physical and sexual abuse. However, Louise did not wish to explore the subject. "I believe in just forgetting about the past and living the best you can. You know what I mean? I don't hold with all this dredging up, playing the victim, blaming your parents. Hey, we all have it hard, don't we? Why whine about it?"

Though I am strongly interested in the psychological aspects of illness, I recognize that psychological work is only an option. It does not always alleviate symptoms, only occasionally produces deep healing, and may awaken deeply buried demons that rise up and cause trouble. Stubborn burial of grief and anger may be the best strategy in certain cases. Anyway, it was Louise's choice, and at this point in our relationship I didn't find it my place to argue.

Still, I couldn't help mentioning that years of battening down the hatches might have caused Louise's chronic muscular tension and headaches. I mentioned this guess gently. She rebuffed me with a disgusted look, and I quickly changed the subject.

We talked about diet and lifestyle. While Louise ate an exemplary, balanced semivegetarian diet, she also admitted to smoking cigarettes. Around this subject, too, she placed a wall, adamantly signaling that she did not wish to change the habit. I obeyed her command.

Louise then questioned me at length for advice about subtle details of her diet. I tried to answer patiently, although I couldn't help thinking that the relative advisability of stir-frying or steaming eggplant rather paled when there were cigarettes to contend with. Nonetheless, I gave her a little advice just to keep her happy.

Later Louise told her friends, "He is the only doctor I know who understands the importance of nutrition."

As for the miracle cure she trumpeted around the city, dramatically lengthening the waiting list of my practice, that occurred during the trial-and-error phase of therapy. First I had to fail with the carefully thought-out treatment I believed would be most helpful.

For twenty-three sessions I performed acupuncture directed toward relaxing her rock-hard sinews. I felt quite confident it would work, for I had been successful with similar problems many times before. To bolster the results I expected, however, I also had her see an expert on movement therapy, who provided Louise with a home exercise program. I also prescribed herbs and nutritional supplements to aid her self-healing abilities.

The net result of this holistic, carefully integrated approach was an absolute lack of improvement. I was frustrated, but Louise continued to grow in enthusiasm. Our dialogues at the beginning of each session would have been amusing to an impartial witness.

"Yes, Dr. Bratman, I really enjoyed the last session. It was a big help." A promising start, but not borne out on questioning.

Q: How was it a help?
A: I felt good, very good after the treatment. I can't get over the fact that you, a medical doctor, are willing to try acupuncture.

Q: Did your neck feel any looser?

A: No, not really.

Q: Did your headaches diminish?

A: Yes! *(I would inflate with anticipation.)* Except I did have four severe headaches and about ten mild ones *(This was the usual number. I would deflate.)* I'm doing much better.

Some alternative physicians, perhaps, can find satisfaction simply in providing the kind of care their patients dream about. Louise certainly felt that her sessions were worthwhile, and she happily signed over her insurance checks to me. But I wanted to see some results. I wanted to justify my income and my time and her insurance company's outlay of cash by actually helping her headaches to improve.

From my point of view, the one good development was that over the course of these fairly fruitless acupuncture hours we developed considerable rapport. I found that I admired this forthright woman for her feisty and potent character. Her stories amazed and educated me. I soon abandoned any covert plans to work the psychological angle. Louise had built an immense and fascinating life on the grounds of forgetting her trauma. Who was I to challenge her philosophy?

Instead I resorted to an emotionally less satisfying but often-times successful method: trying every trick in the book. I tried Japanese, Chinese, Korean, and modern American techniques of acupuncture. I sent her for Feldenkrais, Rolfing, Jin Shin Jyutsu, and chiropractic. I gave her more herbs, vitamins, and even homeo-pathics. I began to lose hope, but Louise felt sure we would succeed.

After six months I suggested she try feverfew, an herb famous for its headache-relieving effects. I had not proposed it earlier be-cause feverfew is mostly used for migraines, and I didn't think she had migraines. Besides, although often quite effective, feverfew is a symptomatic treatment. It doesn't get to the root of the problem at all. Being a good alternative medicine doctor, I didn't want Band-Aid solutions. I wanted to produce real healing. Feverfew did not seem like a great choice. But I was running out of tricks, so I tried it.

Louise had a profound and entirely unexpected reaction to the herb. She came in the following visit looking shocked and amazed. "You're either killing me or curing me!" she said. "But I think you're curing me. That herb you suggested I take—that feverfew?—it's amazing."

When she took the feverfew, Louise explained, the first effect was that she vomited for three hours. She then experienced three times as many hours of diarrhea. Subsequently she was hit with the most intense headache of her life. The whole night she tossed and turned with stabbing pain behind her left eye. For the following four days she suffered a succession of strange and short-lived sensations, from palpitations to partial paralysis to fainting.

"I didn't feel well enough to take a second pill till Friday."

Another patient might have sued me. "My God, Louise, why did you take more after what you went through? You should have called! Don't take feverfew ever again!"

"No, I knew it was all right," she said reassuringly. "I knew it was a healing crisis. I knew I was being cured." Friday night she dreamed a series of intense dreams, roaming through the scenes of her childhood. Over the weekend she felt quite well.

"Today I feel better than I have in years. I'm taking feverfew three times a day now."

I had never expected this. Feverfew, as I know it, is a benign herb. Never before (or since) have I seen it act so explosively. Were I more naïve, I would have leaped to the conclusion that I was onto something big. I might have gone on to write a book titled *The Cure for*

All Headaches! But I had seen it all before. Almost any treatment performs occasional miracles. It's the encores that are so difficult to obtain. I admitted that I had not expected so much from the treatment.

Louise shook her head, smiling. "But you see, Dr. Bratman, you picked just the right herb for me! Maybe it wouldn't do so much for someone else, but for me it was just what I needed. Your intuition led you straight to it."

Straight to it indeed! I was reaching for straws when I wrote down the name.

"You remember when you wanted to play therapist for me?" she continued in a softer voice. "I wouldn't let you, and you were so disappointed. Well, it happened on its own." She paused for effect. "That herb released all my psychological traumas."

I swallowed a few times but did not argue. I just looked at her left eye, wondering how the contraction could have so completely vanished.

A voice inside me said, "It's all the placebo effect, and she's not going to feel better for long." Aloud, I instructed Louise to expect a few ups and downs. "Healing is almost never complete and total all at once," I explained. "It follows a wavelike pattern, with symptoms rising and falling over time. With luck, however, each peak will be lower, each trough shallower, until at last the original symptom will taper away forever." She only chuckled.

To my surprise, the follow-up visits proved little more than opportunities for Louise to praise and pay me. Hers was much more than a temporary or even a wavelike cure. The headaches never returned. What was more, her whole being seemed lighter, as if, without the benefit of psychotherapy, she really had shed the whole weight of her psychic pain.

From that time on I had in Louise a one-woman advertising

team. She told everyone who would listen that I had diagnosed her at a glance, understood her as a whole person, and unerringly prescribed the one substance in the world that could turn her upside down and cure her.

I don't know how to appreciate an experience like this one. The feverfew itself must have been part of it, although in what way I don't understand. The rest was the power of her mind. I hadn't even tried to convince Louise that the feverfew would work. How much more powerful would it have been if I had done a song and dance and presented books, testimonials, persuasive arguments? It was her faith in me that did it, a faith that was due more to her own desires than to my gifts.

I should be grateful for Louise's praise, but I don't feel I can take the credit. The embellished story she tells embarrasses me. At least a dozen patients called me on her direct referral, all expecting a miracle worker. What's worse is that though I produced no miracles, many of these felt their expectations confirmed.

WHAT DOES IT ALL MEAN?

Through experiences like these, as well as my awareness of the complete contradictions between dietary theories, I have grown unimpressed when people tell me stories of their miraculous cures through diet. They speak to me breathlessly; I tap my fingers on the table and wait till they are done.

That is not quite accurate. I am perfectly impressed by the cure, just not by the diet that is supposed to have caused it. I have come to feel that the diet doesn't deserve as much credit as they are giving it. But I feel a kind of kinship toward those diets; I, too, have received undue credit for cures.

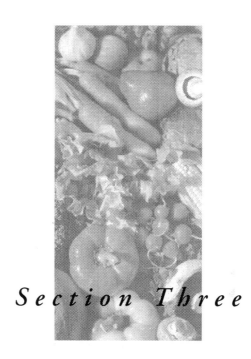

Section Three

RECOVERY

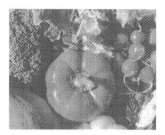

During the research for this book, co-author David Knight posted several articles on orthorexia at selected Web sites. Some of the letters that came back are heartbreaking; all tell of the recognition that orthorexia is an illness and of the desire to escape from bondage.

Have you begun to grow tired of your bondage to healthy diet? Has the ceaseless calculating over meals and crowing over your superiority to others gone flat? Maybe you'd like to be able to share food with friends instead of eating your sprouts alone; perhaps you'd simply like to stop thinking about food so much and get on with your life. This section will help.

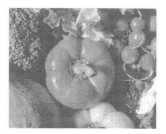

15.

Steps

After reading my magazine articles on orthorexia, many people asked me to explain one sentence that in their view passed too quickly over the most important part of the story. I had written, "It took me at least two more years to attain the ability to follow a middle way in eating easily, without rigid calculation or wild swings."

"But what did you do to get there?" Kathryn asked. "How did you stop feeling guilty over what you ate? How did you stop thinking about food?"

In looking back, I realized that in one matter, at least, I had not told the truth. It took me a lot more than two years. The events described in Chapter 1 occurred in 1979; I can't really say that I relaxed about eating until the early 1990s, more than ten years later. Remembering the wavering course I took and the additional binges into orthorexia I inflicted on myself, my wife, and my children, I recognized a sequence of events in my "recovery." Subsequent interviews with people who have also broken free have shown me that my pattern was fairly typical.

This chapter outlines a series of steps designed to help you break free from orthorexia. In some ways they resemble the twelve steps of AA (although I have taken no efforts to line them up identically). But remember, your chief ally is time. Orthorexia tends to unwind by itself once you admit that you have it; it's nowhere near so powerful as alcoholism or anorexia. Most everyone eventually succeeds.

THE FIRST STEP

As the first step to liberate yourself from the trap of health food obsession, you must admit to yourself that you are trapped and hate it. You need to be able to say, "I am sick of *having* to think about healthy food all the time. I am tired of this obsession. I wish I could go through my life focusing on other things."

Simply admitting this to yourself is surprisingly powerful. It signifies a great change from believing that the way you eat is a mark of your virtue and understanding that it is actually an illness. What is most important is to settle yourself fully in this realization. At first you will find your mind frequently slipping back into its smug interpretations of your eating life. You will hear self-evaluations like "I am such a good person for eating this raw tofu. Look at my in-laws drooling over chicken with barbecue sauce. Oh, what an evolved person I am."

It is important to intensify your awareness that orthorexia is indeed a disease and not a virtue. For some this happens automatically, as time goes on. You begin to loathe your good deeds of eating and to feel increasingly nostalgic for the days when you could have concerns other than your daily menu. As one patient of mine put it, "Once I was aware it was there, the straitjacket started to feel pretty uncomfortable." Over a period of about six months she switched from bragging about her dietary triumphs to speaking of them wearily to sagging with the exhaustion of caring too much about food.

For others an intentional process is helpful. Dana put herself through a formal self-inventory. First she tallied up the harm she had done to others through her fixation on food. The list began as follows:

1. I deprived my daughter of the childhood pleasures of eating ice cream and cake at a birthday party.
2. I gave my mother numerous rather nasty lectures on how badly she had fed me as a child and how badly she was eating today.
3. I even kept my daughter from staying over at her grandmother's because I knew she'd eat cookies and drink milk.
4. I allowed myself to become estranged from my good friend Barbara by acting superior over a matter of white-flour pasta.

As Dana continued to work with it, the list grew to forty entries. At the same time she worked on making amends to those she felt she had harmed, surprising her friends and relatives by calling up at odd hours to apologize for "laying dietary guilt trips on you."

Besides harming others, of course, orthorexia harms the orthorexic herself badly. Dana's list of how she had hurt herself included the following:

1. For seven years I spent more than half my waking time obsessing over food. I never took the watercolor classes I'd promised myself. I never relaxed and really enjoyed myself

when I was with friends. I stopped going backpacking because I couldn't carry my foods with me.

2. I spent years in an obnoxious state of self-congratulation, which, now that I think about it, poisoned my soul.

3. I lied to myself about how much I enjoyed the tasteless foods that I permitted myself to eat, which got me started lying to myself about lots of other things, too.

4. I turned down several friendships and relationships that could have meant a lot to me, over food snobbery.

This list, too, grew in length, reaching about thirty entries. Dana would hold it in her hand and feel the heft of it whenever she forgot. "It is evidence, hard evidence," she would say. "I use the list to remind myself that I'm not falling *off* the path of righteousness as I work to free myself from orthorexia. 'Cause it always feels that I'm doing something wrong, even though I know what I'm doing is right. When the raw grains beckon to me, I hold up the list and say, 'No! Keep away. See what you've done to me? You're not good the way you pretend. You're a temptation I have to resist.' "

Charles used a similar method. Working together, we created affirmations to remind him of his right to find a different way to live. "Life is too short to spend it obsessing over food" was his favorite. He made a bumper sticker out of it and looked at it when he felt like wavering. "It's tangible, something actually stuck to the bumper of my car," he would say. "It has to be true; it's in print."

He also liked to say, as a mantra, "My mind belongs to me, not to my vegetables." Another phrase that worked very well for him was the paradoxical "If I spend more than an hour a day thinking about food, I'm a bad person." I'm not sure I'd recommend this particular affirmation to most people, as it could certainly backfire and make you feel bad about yourself. But for Charles its value was its shock effect, reversing the interior programming that always said "If I *don't* think constantly about food, I'm a bad person."

For me the awareness that I was harming myself first came in a dream about tomatoes. In late spring of 1977 I had helped plant baby tomato plants, about four hundred of them, and plunged stakes into the ground nearby. Every week I would rototill up and down the rows, keeping out the weeds without using any pesticides. When the tomatoes were big enough, I spent a full day tying them to the stakes, using a special soft twist tie recommended for the purpose. You had to tie them tight enough to keep the plants from falling over but loose enough to allow them to live. It was a bit of an art, and I obsessed quite a lot about whether I was doing it right.

The night after the tying I dreamed about those tomatoes. In the dream I had tied all the plants too tightly. They were trying to grow against the restraint of the twist ties but were unable to break out. The wires dug deeper and deeper into the flesh of their stems. The tomato plants responded by forming a callus, but it wasn't strong enough, and the wire bit in ever more deeply. In the dream I tried to loosen the wire, but it was too late, and the plants were keeling over in their rows, their life force blocked off by the squeezing pressure of the too-tight ties.

I didn't need an official dream analysis to understand this one. I was being too strict with myself. I was tying myself too tightly, in the supposed interest of health, blocking the flow of my own life. I knew I had to loosen up. Although it was years before I could make a change, I held on to the dream the way Dana grasped her lists or Charles his affirmations. It was something tangible. It burned this message into my brain: "Your eating is not a virtue. It's a problem."

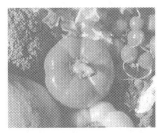

16.

Identifying
Hidden Agendas

After thoroughly admitting to yourself that you are sick and tired of your obsession with healthy food, the next step is to identify the reasons you became obsessed in the first place. It will be a lot easier to break free if you know what's holding you back. It may be that you only wanted to eat healthier and simply took it too far. But as I described in Chapter 5, there are often a number of hidden agendas involved.

To recap, these are:

Illusion of Total Safety: The false belief that you can completely prevent illness by eating right.

This fantasy whispers, "You will never die so long as you avoid junk food." And, conversely, "One french fry will bring death just around the corner."

Get real. Death is much more powerful than you are. You can perhaps keep it away for a bit longer (on a statistical average) by eating properly, but we're only talking percentages.

Desire for Complete Control: Using the tiny world of food to convince yourself that your whole life is under your control.

You can focus all your angst on the important question of how best to slice the carrots and thereby avoid unpleasant subjects such as "What am I doing with my life anyway?" However, since your life can never really be under complete control, this is a form of playing pretend. In any case, it's boring. Life's chaos and unpredictability are what make it better than a novel or a Shakespeare play. You can't really iron out the unexpected twists and surprising accidents anyway. You *can* achieve absolute control over what enters your mouth, if you are so inclined, and have the will and the middle- or upper-class means to afford it. But it's demeaning. Rather than be the master of such a small realm, why not participate in a larger and more chaotic world?

Covert Conformity: Using healthy diet as a way to pursue the Barbie ideal without admitting it to yourself.

Do you secretly enjoy the fact that your special foods keep you thin? Would you never admit to dieting for that purpose but enjoy receiving it as a kind of side effect? Be honest with yourself. If you are under the spell of society's beliefs about weight, admit it to yourself, and then decide exactly how much you want that expectation to rule you.

Searching for Spirituality in the Kitchen: Using food as a primary source of spiritual satisfaction.

The problem is that food is too narrow an object to fulfill your spiritual needs. Find other ways to connect spiritually with the world, through nature, meditation, a spiritual group, singing. Expand your soul to the sky rather than contracting it to lentil size.

Food Puritanism: Using food restrictions as a form of asceticism, delighting in denying yourself the fulfillment of your desires.

Do you like punishing yourself? Ascetics in many parts of the world have engaged in practices to mortify the flesh, whether flagellating themselves, sleeping on a bed of nails, or eating nothing but stale bread. Denying yourself the gluttonous desires of the body might help you find a life in the spirit. If you wish to torture yourself in this way, then by all means go for it. But be honest. Don't pretend that you simply prefer to eat nothing but brown rice. And if you really enjoy depriving yourself, more than just as a means to an end, perhaps you should see a psychotherapist.

Creating an Identity: Giving yourself a place in the world in terms of food.

This was one of my prime motivations for becoming orthorexic. I couldn't bear to be simply one of the masses; I had to stand out in some way. My complicated dietary rules gave me a name and an identity. They also nicely separated me from others. Furthermore, by being a raw foods vegetarian, I had a ready-made community with a shared sense of values when I wanted it.

I eventually decided that food wasn't a creative enough focus to build an identity around. It was a good stepping-stone to finding myself, but I had to grow out of it someday.

Fear of Other People: Using a severe food trip as a way to avoid socially uncomfortable situations.

If you are afraid of other people, needing to consume your specially prepared barley sprout juice is a great excuse for not getting out. I used to relish my yogurt with raw nuts and strawberries and chew it so slowly in my room that by the time I was done, all my housemates were gone.

Of course, there's nothing wrong with privacy. If you want to be alone, be alone. But don't pretend you just want to chew your food in peace. It's the self-dishonesty that is the disease here, the corrupting pretense that you are making choices for one reason while really following a different agenda.

STORIES

For Dana the obvious hidden agenda was a sense of identity. She had grown up in a fringe Christian group that amounted to a cult. Although she had escaped from it years before and found her way to a more mainstream form of Christianity, somewhere inside she missed the extreme rigors of her early practice and the way it set her above the rest of the world. She had first become a macrobiotic adherent to improve her health. However, soon the older drives plugged in, and she used macrobiotics to reinstate the old, comfortable feelings.

Once she realized this, Dana knew what she needed to do. "I used the same tricks that helped me get out of the cult. I reminded myself that feeling better than other people is actually anti-Christian. You're not supposed to separate yourself from other people. You're supposed to feel that everyone is your sister or brother. Besides, the Bible never says, 'Thou shalt despise those who eat the wrong things.' Actually, Jesus said something like 'It isn't what goes into your mouth that defiles you but what comes out of it.' He wouldn't have been very happy to hear me slandering people over what they eat. It hurt to admit this to myself, but it helped me more than anything."

Charles found help with his orthorexia when he saw a psychotherapist. "She showed me the unconscious beliefs at work inside me. To say it simply, I felt that I deserved to be punished. If I wanted something, that desire had to be evil. It wasn't just with food, but food was the easiest place to see it.

"The story goes like this: I started by cutting out fatty foods because I was a little overweight, and my cholesterol was a bit on the high side. But it just kept on escalating. I'd hate myself for weeks if I ate the wrong vegetable or drank too much liquid with my meals. It seemed that no matter how healthy my diet became, I would always raise the bar higher, just for the pleasure, almost, of seeing myself fall."

Although he didn't call it that, Charles had noticed his own food puritanism for years. At first he saw it as just "worrying too much." He tried to let go and relax. But it didn't work. Food had a huge grip on him.

Only when the force of his interior habit became clear did Charles finally decide to see a therapist. There he began to understand the hidden agenda that kept him orthorexic. It wasn't merely that he worried too much. He was caught up in a more complex tangle of emotions and needed to take more specific steps.

On the therapist's advice Charles pasted affirmations all over his house that read, "I am a good person. I have a right to enjoy myself."

"At first I just couldn't believe any of it," he says. "Whenever I'd read those affirmations, a little voice in my head would say, 'No you don't. You don't deserve anything.'"

However, as the work he did in therapy began to pay off, Charles found himself increasingly able to "take in" the messages he was putting up. His orthorexia actually slipped away by itself over subsequent months.

Kathy was caught up in the illusion of absolute control. She did not initially come to me for treatment of orthorexia. Quite the contrary. On my intake form she wrote, "I need help eating more strictly."

Kathy was an adherent of macrobiotics and had been for many years. However, she felt that she had lingering health problems due to her occasional episodes of "cheating." She wanted me to help her follow the strictest possible macrobiotic diet.

When I first saw Kathy, I was struck by the unhealthy look of her auburn/gray hair. It looked dry, brittle, well matched to the dull skin of her face. Her voice fit in well, too, sounding rigid and bitten out, although quiet, perhaps like that of a drill sergeant with laryngitis.

Kathy's problem, as she understood it, was that she habitually abandoned the brown rice so central to macrobiotics and ate wheat instead.

"I love wheat, but it makes my stomach hurt," she said.

"How tender does it get?" I asked. "Put it on a scale of one to ten, where ten is the worst pain you've ever experienced and one is a little scratch."

She thought about it. "I'd say it's maybe a four."

"Can you put it out of your mind by getting busy?" I asked.

She agreed that she could. "Okay, maybe it's a three," she admitted.

"Does it wake you at night?"

"No," she said. "I supposed you'd call it a two. But if I push real hard right here, it's uncomfortable."

My first thought was that most people will hurt in the stomach when they push "real hard." But I didn't say anything.

She looked contrite. "I know I should just give up wheat entirely, but it's hard. Sometimes I . . ." Her voice cracked slightly. "Sometimes I crave bread, and then I'll buy some and eat it with olive oil on it." She looked both sad and guilty now. I knew that I was supposed to shake my head and cluck, to say, "How can you ever expect to feel well if you insist on indulging in the evil of bread?"

But I said nothing and just looked at her. Suddenly she brightened and offered, "Maybe there's some herb I could take so I could get away with eating wheat. I really like to eat it."

That sounded like an improvement to me, better at least than feeling guilty about a desire for wheat. Although I didn't think that what Kathy really needed most was to put something else into her mouth, I decided to take this suggestion as someplace to start. I wrote out a recommendation for a few digestive herbs and asked her to come back in a week.

When Kathy returned, she looked as sad as ever. "I'm so bad," she said, shaking her head, her long brittle hair brushing her knees.

"What did you do?" I asked. "Sell drugs to elementary school students? Burn down a church? Sell your niece into slavery?"

That provoked the first real smile I'd seen from her. "No, nothing like that. What I did was eat cheddar cheese." She hung her head. "I'm so undisciplined that way." She said the word "undisciplined" with a kind of bitter passion. "I just don't have any discipline. At least once a month I eat something I shouldn't."

No discipline! Kathy had enough self-discipline to make Mahatma Gandhi jealous (he slipped up on his vows from time to time, too). But I had to approach this delicately or risk losing her trust.

"Kathy," I said, "I take a different view. In my opinion your slipups are a desperate attempt by your good sense to restore balance."

Again she smiled fleetingly. "But macrobiotics is all about balance. I have to balance my foods, and if I don't, I get sick."

"You mean, you get punished for enjoying yourself," I said, and once more saw the smile that showed me I was on the right track. "In Asian medicine, of which, as you know, macrobiotics is a part, too much self-control is an imbalance in itself. Excessive self-strictness is believed to produce what is called a liver imbalance. It leads to numerous symptoms, among them crampy abdominal pain."

That was the right angle, and also true. Her face lit up thoughtfully. "You mean that by trying so hard, I'm actually making myself sicker?"

It was a start. Over the next nineteen months we worked together closely. Kathy found it extremely difficult to get away from her self-imposed strictness. It seemed to her that habits developed in a rather punitive upbringing had transferred over to food. She easily felt guilty, in the wrong, deserving of punishment. Whenever she felt any spontaneous impulse, she instinctively suppressed it. The only environment that felt right to her was a strict, completely controlled one, without any room for spontaneity or free expression.

Eventually Kathy hit on an original solution to her problem: She took up improvisational theater. Its emphasis on free expression of emotion proved liberating. On the stage she let go of her strict self-control. Her voice grew more audible and eventually even loud, its monotone modulated into a range of expression.

What's more, in time the new ability to express emotion carried over into her real life. She no longer felt the need to strictly regulate her diet. Nonetheless, she still ate healthy food—just not insanely healthy. And with her greater range of feeling came an increased ability to digest as well. It was as if she had increased all the energy within herself and didn't have to be so finicky.

• • •

Orthorexia is really a lot easier to overcome than other major addictions, such as alcoholism or compulsive gambling. While it is rare that psychotherapy or improvisational theater alone would succeed for these conditions, orthorexia will often start to fall away by itself once you take the first two steps, acknowledging that it exists and then unraveling the hidden agendas that give it extra power. But another issue may then arise: How should you eat?

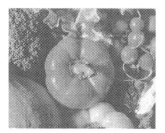

17.

Eating Healthy Without Obsession: Finding the Middle Way

Once you have accepted that you have orthorexia and have decided to eat more normally, you still have to learn how to do it. You have disciplined yourself to do something quite extreme. Learning how to follow a middle path and to do so naturally, without thinking about it too much, can be quite difficult and sometimes even hilarious.

When I first came to realize that I had orthorexia, I thought I could just break out of it by deciding to do so. I would set down the heavy burden of planning, obsession, and the pursuit of dietary perfection and instead eat in a generally healthful way.

I made this decision in the evening (about a week after my ice cream binge), and I had no problem with the resolution until morning came. Then I had to decide what to eat for breakfast. I didn't know how to eat without thinking intensely about it. My head had ruled my appetite for so long that I couldn't hear my stomach. How could I prepare a breakfast without carefully considering it first? How could I decide how much to eat at a meal without debating which foods should take the largest places on my plate?

Seeing nothing on my own shelves but excessively healthy food (raw millet and the like), I bravely drove off in search of a restaurant where I could pursue my return to normal dietary life. The first restaurant I saw was Denny's. Although I went so far as to turn into the parking lot, I continued on through to the far exit, unwilling to take a dive off such a high cliff. Next I drove around looking for a wholesome little place, the sort with flowers painted on the outside walls, serving food that, although edible, would be at least reasonably healthy. I reasoned that to try to eat at Denny's would be to go too far in the other direction, and I congratulated myself on seeking the middle way.

Unfortunately, I couldn't find any restaurants with flowers painted on the walls. I saw truck stops, diners, and chains not much different from Denny's; in a brief spurt of reckless heroism I circled around a McDonald's. But having not eaten at restaurants for several years, I wasn't capable of homing in on the type I now wanted. I became unsure whether I had ever even seen such a restaurant or whether I was remembering a scene from a movie. Maybe it was a past life. In any case, I was starting to feel quite hungry and a bit faint. I stopped to look in a phone book, but the restaurant pages were torn out. I found another phone book, but the only advertisement that seemed remotely correct described a café clear across town. I needed sustenance more rapidly.

In desperation I considered eating Chinese food for breakfast, but backed off out of fear of MSG. I finally turned into the parking lot of a supermarket and decided to forage among the raw ingredients of normal food.

I think I had a vague plan of cooking whole-wheat pancakes. But when I found only white-flour pancake mix and fake maple syrup, my hand faltered. I then discovered oatmeal and rushed with it to the cashier. At the last moment I realized it was instant oatmeal, a food that clearly couldn't have much in the way of life force, and mumbling some incoherent explanation, I returned it to the shelf. I came back a moment later hugging the real oatmeal to my side, only to further confuse the clerk by stopping to read its label, then going back in search of butter and brown sugar.

I finally came home in a frenzy of mixed thoughts and considerable hunger. I felt guilty over all my indecision, which clearly contradicted my goal of eating without obsession, and at the same time I felt a strong need to avoid the brown sugar. But it said "add butter and brown sugar" right there in the label instructions, and if I wanted to eat like a normal person, I would have to join in.

I cooked the oatmeal for a shorter period than recommended, in order to keep as much life force in as possible, and then added about an eighth of a teaspoon of butter and still less brown sugar. A few bites later this seemed like cheating, so I added some more of each and then felt so disgusted by the sweetness that I threw it out and made some more. Eventually I ate enough oatmeal to feel sick, which led me to fast for the rest of the day. Apparently I hadn't solved the transition problem quite yet.

I decided next to take a first, intermediate step before leaping off into the world of normal eating. I would serve myself large portions of the foods I had previously focused upon, such as raw vegetables, and add only small amounts of standard American fare, such as cheese. But as soon as I tried that, I recognized that I was calculating again, so in defiance of my orthorexia I took a second serving of cheese—this time far too much, leading to a stomachache and fasting again.

Actually, I'm not even sure if I really had a stomachache. Maybe it was just the sensation of fullness that seemed wrong after I'd come to appreciate lightness in the belly. But it seemed like a stomachache.

After fasting I'd feel so hungry that I'd gorge myself again and wind up eating a meal of fruit alone, to let my stomach rest. I seemed to have lost the ability to tell whether I'd eaten enough or too little, which made it difficult to navigate between hunger and overeating. It was like bulimia in some ways, only I wasn't at all concerned about my weight. It was like anorexia, too, in that I was so attached to the feeling of lightness that comes with eating little. But it was neither of these. It was orthorexia refusing to let go without a struggle.

Meanwhile, I was now able to notice fellow members of the commune who were similarly afflicted. One man in his early twenties would fill his plate with mounds of peanut butter and raw wheat berries and eye it with a kind of self-loathing before digging in. A woman in her forties would serve herself a tureen of lettuce; I thought she looked like a rabbit eating it. I'd peer at my own plate and wonder how it looked to others; I'd surreptitiously examine the plates of those I regarded as normal eaters and try to copy what I found there. I found myself reading nutrition books to learn how an average serving of a particular food was typically defined.

Finally I hit on the notion of "the plate" and "the bowl." This technique involved filling a single plate or bowl with normal serving sizes of the constituents of a balanced meal. Then I would allow myself seconds on any one food. I figured that by using this method I would neither starve nor fill my stomach to the point of pain. I later found that some dieters used the same method, but to avoid gaining weight. For me, the method helped give me bounds on what eating should be like and set a limit on my culinary cogitation.

Subsequently I have met other people who found similar solutions. Charlotte religiously followed recipe plans in books, refusing to make any allowances for what she liked or didn't like in order to avoid getting into confusion about it. Ellen asked friends to tell her what to eat, and when that well dried up, she started designing meals weeks in advance and religiously sticking to her decisions. Gary resolved to eat perfectly most of the time, but on weekends he would eat out and accept whatever was served at a friend's house, at a restaurant, or by his mother.

The most important principle is to take slow and gentle steps toward eating like a moderate person again. The meals you choose should be reasonably healthy, because if you try to eat junk food, you'll feel excessive guilt. However, the meals shouldn't be "perfect" according to your previous standards, or you won't get anywhere. You have to work on breaking up your extremism one step at a time.

Keep in mind that you might feel a few physical symptoms, whether from the actual imperfection of the food or from your imagination it's hard to say. "I feel so awful when I eat heavy food," one recovering raw foods vegetarian complained. It's true; if you switch from raw foods to normal food, you won't feel like a transparent angel of light tripping through life as an animated sunbeam. You'll feel like a person, with some heaviness, some lightness. Your skin won't feel like "an energy membrane connecting you to life" but like skin, a little oily perhaps, or a little dry. Your stomach will feel at times as if it has food in it, and your abdomen will do some work and make some noise. Sometimes you'll feel energetic, and sometimes you'll feel tired. From time to time you'll get sick. You'll fart or burp occasionally. In short, you'll be a normal person. You are neither perfect nor depraved. Just human.

This decision requires acceptance of the heaviness and folly that goes along with living a normal life, keeping firmly in mind that the key to health is balance, not extremism. Aristotle called it the Golden Mean.

For her first step Carol used a method I called Intentional Exceptions. She was a food allergy fanatic, and for her, healing orthorexia meant deliberately "cheating" on her diet. She started with one cheat a week and then worked up to one violation a day. At first she developed annoying physical symptoms, like muscle aches and blurry vision, but after a while they stopped. "My body is starting to tolerate more foods," she said after three months of diligent cheating.

Of course, if you are a true orthorexic, these suggestions will sound like heresy. "Eat food I'm allergic to? Have an ice cream cone once a month? You might as well ask me to rob a convenience store. It's out of the question." But you have to let go of dietary perfection if you want to break free from orthorexia. You have to stop caring so fervently about what you eat. Yes, by all means eat a *generally* healthy diet. Just not a *perfectly* healthy diet.

UNWINDING

But no matter how slowly you take it, it isn't easy for an orthorexic to relax about eating. Can a pack-a-day smoker casually forget his cigarettes for a weekend? The obsession of orthorexia has to be unwound slowly and gradually. You should anticipate flare-ups of increased obsession alternating with small advances, strange reactive behavior that carries you through mood changes, and peculiar dietary choices that don't fit any theory known to man. There is no shortcut that bypasses these peregrinations. You have to live through it, remembering that time is your ally. The twists and turns will gradually smooth out, and things will get easier for you.

The most important thing is to go easy on the guilt. Condemning yourself for oversteering to the junk side or the other way to the obsessively healthy side will only complicate your recovery. Under the pressure of guilt you'll just get more obsessive. Remember the image of the tomato plant. You have to loosen up a bit, and that includes giving yourself space to make some mistakes. Eventually the impossible will become habitual: You'll eat a generally healthy diet without freaking out about it.

VISITING YOUR MOTHER

One of your biggest tests as a recovering orthorexic is to go to your mother's house and eat graciously. The usual complications regarding one's parents combine with food obsession to create a special level of insanity. I vividly recall visiting my own mother during the delicate period of leaving orthorexia behind. It was with a great sense of saintly virtue that I planned to indulge her imposition on my health. Before starting, I went to the bathroom and there took a vow to eat what she served me. But when I sat down to a table heaped with the food I had grown up on, I nearly had a panic attack. I have to admit that what she served called to me with a sense of underlying comfort, but this complicated the issue, because I didn't want to admit that I was still fond of food that didn't jibe with my beliefs. Iceberg lettuce (good heavens, no nutrients!) salad with raw mushrooms ("rotten" food according to the theory I had most recently followed), and chopped carrots (better, but unwholesome if eaten raw), canned split pea soup (lacking in life force), garlic French bread (with Kraft cheese). I scarcely noticed that she had catered to me so far as to make me something vegetarian, so full of scorn was I for the violations of my eating beliefs.

I carefully examined all the jars of salad dressing on the lazy Susan, trying to choose the lesser of many evils. Eventually I settled on a vinaigrette. (I considered asking her for plain oil and vinegar to avoid the preservatives in the premade dressing, but that would have violated my rule of accepting what was before me.) The soup caused me the fewest problems, although I couldn't forbear lecturing my mother on the virtues of purchasing organic split peas and cooking soup from scratch, rather than serving canned soup. But the French bread gave me feelings of betrayal; with the Kraft cheese and white flour it seemed artificial to the nth degree, from my point of view a type of middle-grade plastic. I imagined chunks of artificial cheese-colored material collecting like amber in my gut; I saw it lining my digestive tract and, together with the lumps of white flour, interfering with the absorption of any healthful nutrients.

I went to the bathroom again and said aloud seven times, "I will accept this food because it is offered to me. I will accept this food because it is offered to me." I came back out still saying it, and against the pressure of this inner mantra my ability to carry on a normal conversation was sharply limited. I found myself criticizing the preservatives in the dressing, the mushrooms in the salad, and the artificially flavored fruit drink in the cups, combining the superiority of an orthorexic with the insulting manners toward one's parents so common in children of the sixties.

I do not look back on that evening with anything but shame. How could I have been so ungracious, so arrogant, so self-centered? But I did it again dozens of times before I could behave in a way that I don't cringe to recall.

EATING A SPECIAL DIET WITHOUT ORTHOREXIA

Reading the above, you might conclude that I believe that eating a certain proportion of junk food is the most desirable outcome in life. But actually that isn't my message at all. There's nothing wrong with eating healthfully, and there's a lot right to it. The problem is not the nature of the diet itself but your attitude toward it. It is the obsession with food, the inability to drop the issue when appropriate (such as when you are eating at your mother's house), the failure to maintain a sense of proportion that turns healthy eating into orthorexia. If you can eat food that makes you feel good or that you believe will prevent illness, that's wonderful. The point is to do it in a relaxed way, remembering that there is more to life than eating.

The major issue is, Are you a fanatic? Do you think about food all the time? Do you have trouble not thinking about it? If you can eat a diet without thinking about it too much, you are probably not orthorexic. Gandhi ate mostly fruits and nuts for periods of his life. Clearly he was not solely obsessed with eating; he had a few other things on his plate besides food.

There are many good reasons to adopt a special diet. Perhaps you have developed ethical scruples against eating meat and want to be a pure vegetarian. Or you may have a serious illness and find that avoiding allergenic foods makes you feel fabulously better. Similarly, your best understanding of the scientific evidence might lead you to believe that largely limiting your diet to grains, vegetables, and tofu is the best route to long life and continued good health. All these reasons, and others besides, well justify adopting a carefully selected diet. The question is, Can you eat according to special rules without becoming orthorexic?

Of course you can. There is actually no contradiction between eating a healthy diet and avoiding the eating disorder of orthorexia. It's just tricky. One of the trickiest parts is that the emotions appropriate for starting a diet can lead to orthorexia if they remain unchanged over time.

THE FIRST MONTHS OF A NEW DIET

A certain amount of fanaticism is necessary in the beginning. It is very difficult to alter one's diet, and in order to get started, you might have to work up a head of steam.

During the first months of a new diet you are homesick for junk food, you long for the sense of comfort and familiarity that goes along with it. The image of a favored meal—a pizza, for example, with a tall beer—floats before your mind like home at the end of a long trip. You long to settle down at a familiar table, eating your familiar food, putting aside the feeling of sojourning and drinking the comfort of the known. In those early days of dietary change there is the constant risk of breaking out of your diet and then, finding the comfort irresistible, not returning again for weeks. Your original food seems to satisfy the mouth more, fill the stomach, and generally feel like an actual meal rather than a dose of medicine.

Often the only solution to temptation is to get really excited about your diet, even to the point of irrationality, and to exercise iron discipline to avoid falling off the path. This may annoy your friends, yet at the same time it may be the only path toward your goal. I don't call it orthorexia if you are only six months into a diet, or less, and behave like one who is obsessed. It's only natural.

A YEAR LATER

Initially, a certain amount of dietary fanaticism is understandable. But if a year into a diet you are still rigid and psychologically possessed, you are starting to have a problem. Eventually you need to find a way of eating well without obsessing over it.

With the right attitude you can probably succeed at relaxing. You need to keep in mind that your goal is to drop the fanaticism once you've succeeded at making the change. If you hold this thought at the back of your mind from the very beginning, you will find that the extremism you need to start a food religion will wear off as it becomes easier to follow its rules without effort. You will no longer fear that the slightest deviation from the rules will lead to a spiral of "cheating," because your new way of eating will have become habitual to you.

The big ally in this process is time. If you eat tofu long enough, it will begin to feel comforting on its own. After all, dietary patterns are just habits. It is initially difficult to change the habits of a lifetime, to eat tofu instead of burgers, but once you have done so for a season or two, the tofu tastes good and the amount of self-discipline you need decreases dramatically. The healthy diet you've chosen will also be satisfying to the tongue and stomach. You will find it comforting. It will have become home.

You reach a point where you don't really have to worry so much about falling off the wagon. You *can* eat a meat loaf served by a friend, because it *won't* set you going on a binge of junk food. Burgers will start to seem like a type of food rather than the mystically attractive forbidden fruit they seemed in the early days of your dietary change. They will taste okay, but perhaps a little greasy.

The important consideration here is to withdraw your mind gradually from the act of eating. If you make a whole mental production over the notion that a burger is toxic poison, if you dwell on the idea that it is dripping with unholy grease and is rotting every lymph node in your body, you will produce the reverse effect in the subterranean layers of your heart. The more you claim to hate it, the more you will inwardly idealize it. The more you claim it makes you sick, the more it will represent pleasure denied. You will sneak out in the night to buy a burger, with all the passion of a forbidden love affair. The secret self that feels deprived and in moments of weakness cries "I deserve a break from the discipline! I deserve to be indulged!" will focus its ardor on burgers, and you will live out the common dance of orthorexia: fanatically pursuing certain foods during the day and shamefully sneaking the opposite at night. (Of course, never will a burger taste so good as when you sneak one in defiance of your diet. It is almost worth being half crazed to appreciate the gourmet subtleties of bad food.)

Another helpful rule is to make sure not to tell your friends about the merits of your diet and all the diseases you hope it will prevent. Talk about movies, talk about children, talk about politics. If your brain says, "I must preach to my friends so that they can feel as great as I do," counter with "Fine, but wait for a year." New converts to anything are simply annoying if they can't help talking about their beloved beliefs. Wait until your discovery has settled (meaning that you still believe in it a year or two later) before you hold block parties to evangelize. Not only will this help you keep your friends, it will encourage you to treat diet as an ordinary rather than an extraordinary feature of life.

On the same principle, while you are eating, refrain from studying books about your diet or feverishly planning your next meal. Do everything you can to enjoy yourself in an ordinary manner so you can remember the moment with ordinary pleasure. It's much safer and saner.

The last rule to keep in mind is rather subtle and difficult, and you may require the assistance of a psychotherapist if it trips you up. This involves noticing when hidden agendas creep in, and saying no. For example, if you find yourself feeling decidedly superior to other people who don't eat the way you do, you have to find a way to throw that pernicious thought out of your brain. Or if you catch yourself dealing with an anxious moment in some other aspect of your life by thinking about your great diet, you are using diet as an escape, and it will trap you. Review Chapter 16 for any other hidden agendas, and if you recognize yourself in any of them, get help. Otherwise the chances are slim that your diet will only improve health; it will insidiously turn into orthorexia.

Diet needs to be just diet, not a means for creating isolation, control, or self-punishment. If you can keep this in perspective, you'll do fine.

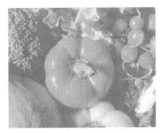

18.

For Friends and Health Care Professionals: When to Intervene

Although extreme diets may appear crazy to an insider, individuals clearly have a right to make choices. I may feel that it makes no sense to focus obsessively on food, considering the other ways to spend one's time, but who am I to make this decision for someone else? If a person wants to collect stamps, run for political office, or join a strict religion, I may find any of these choices disagreeable, but I don't have a right to stop that person.

However, there are times when by consensus most of us would say that intervention makes sense, for example, with alcoholism, severe depression, and anorexia. This chapter addresses the confusing question of when it is appropriate to intervene in the life of a health food fanatic.

EASY DECISIONS

I had no problem deciding that Morgan needed help. Over the course of three years he had wandered into a diet so restrictive I didn't know how long he would survive. A quick analysis of his diet showed that it contained less than 5 percent of the amount of protein someone his size would need daily and next to no calories at all. He looked terrible, he weighed less than a hundred pounds, and I knew he was a sitting duck for major infection.

Morgan had started out as a standard raw-foodist but had progressively narrowed his food intake to allow only vegetables; he ate no grains or legumes, and the few vegetables that might have tided him over, such as potatoes, were off-limits because he did not believe in cooking. He discounted the warnings of his few remaining friends, because he thought he knew better, but he obviously wasn't thriving. In my opinion he was fooling himself, rather than following a higher dietary calling. It's not that he was trying to kill himself. He had just wrapped his mind around extremist theories so completely that he'd lost all sense of balance.

Wanting to keep his goodwill, I tried various tricks I'd used successfully on other occasions, such as attempting to interest him in more livable although equally fanatical food trips. But it didn't work. He kept going mournfully forward, certain that he was doing the right thing, while deepening his malnutrition.

I finally enlisted the aid of his sister and had him hospitalized against his will. For a long time he hated me for it, but a year later he admitted that I'd done him a favor.

On the other side of the coin, I had very little doubt that I should not take any drastic steps with Mary. In fact, I couldn't see any justification even for trying to push her gently in another direction.

Mary was a devout macrobiotics follower, whose every minute was spent in contemplation of food. She had few friendships, little ambition in life, and no outside interests. But she was happy in her little macrobiotic world. What's more, I knew her past history. Mary had been badly abused as a child, and up until her discovery of macrobiotics her life had veered from one disaster to another. The rigid culture of her dietary faith seemed to be just what the doctor ordered. I would have regarded any suggestion to try to change her attitude as an act of deliberate cruelty.

Even when diet doesn't seem to be a necessary psychological crutch, it is generally quite impertinent to try to "fix" a problem in another person who hasn't asked for your help. Just as orthorexics can be quite obnoxious about evangelizing their food beliefs to others, those who do not believe much in diet can just as obnoxiously find it their duty to disparage those who do. In my opinion you should not make any comment about someone's dietary habits unless requested to, or if you perceive one of the five situations I describe later in the chapter.

THE GRAY ZONE

With Alice, I wasn't at all sure how to regard her fixation on diet. She had become a raw foods vegetarian after a painful divorce. It seemed to me that she found in raw-foodism a chance to avoid facing life; the quest for lightness and closeness to the plant kingdom seemed to me to hide a considerable element of escape. If it were up to me, I'd suggest that she find a way to face her disappointment, rather than run away from it.

But the way she managed her raw foods diet was certainly healthy. And if someone wants to run away from life rather than face it, what business is it of mine to argue? She had every right to seek the world of the spirit and reject the earth, even if she did so through the medium of food rather than conventional spirituality. Everyone has avocations and makes choices. A professional basketball player or a great physicist is escaping just as much of life as a raw-foodist.

Becoming a raw foods fanatic is a choice, like other choices. It closes some possibilities while opening others. It is both noble and ignoble, brave and cowardly, like many life choices. So I decided to do nothing and say nothing and simply appreciate her as any other eccentric character.

At least until she began proselytizing to one of my other patients.

PROSELYTIZING

Sixteen-year-old Cynthia ran into Alice at a health fair and found the message of raw-foodism compelling. She came to an appointment full of enthusiasm for her new discovery.

"This woman explained to me that unless you eat foods raw, they don't have any enzymes and don't keep you healthy. She really impressed me. She says raw foods are her whole life, and I thought it was really cool."

From the way Cynthia described her, I quickly recognized Alice. While I had no objection to Alice's pursuing her extreme raw foods lifestyle, I felt an obligation to give Cynthia a more rounded message. It's one matter to make a radical decision for yourself, another to convince others to join you. In the latter case I believe that friends and health care professionals have a right and perhaps an obligation to tell the other side of the story.

I explained to Cynthia that the enzyme part of raw foods theory was probably all wrong and, more important, that the altered state raw-foodism creates is exciting, but it's also kind of an escape from life. "In a way it's like taking psychedelics," I said. "It definitely gives you some ecstatic feelings, but in a way it cheats you out of really living on earth."

All's fair in love and food theories. I clinched the deal by mentioning another issue close to Cynthia's heart, one that I found more sane and balanced. "Native Americans weren't raw-foodists. Oh, sure, they might fast for a vision quest or some such specific purpose, and I have no disagreement with that, but most of the time they were really grounded. They didn't try to fly away—they lived here, on earth. I think it's actually much more real to be a person than to try to be an angel."

There are many lifestyle choices that I accept in those who have adopted them but would argue against when those people begin to evangelize. Individuals have a right to their own opinions, but my friends and clients have a right to my opinions, too, along with the other opinions they receive.

WHEN TO DRAW THE LINE

There are five circumstances in which I start to think about taking action with a patient who is obsessed with healthy food. Of course, each of these is a judgment call, but each seems to me like a situation in which a judgment really has to be made.

1. When a diet goes past the point of safety
2. When a diet seems to be making a person miserable

3. When someone admits that he or she would like to quit an extreme diet but can't
4. When it seems that a third party is involved, creating what amounts to a dietary cult
5. When a diet seems to have become an emotional illness

When a diet goes past the point of safety

Although breatharians believe they can live on no food at all, most of us would consider them to be deluded. If a person isn't getting very much in the way of protein or total calories, I think it's pretty clear that that person is not taking good care of him- or herself. In such situations it is just as appropriate to intervene as it would in the case of an elderly person who isn't eating or a depressed person who isn't getting out of bed. Those who have fallen for bizarre dietary theories may need outside help, whether they ask for it or not. In such cases it may be the duty of a friend or health care professional to take steps.

When a diet seems to be making a person miserable

Sometimes it is painfully obvious that a person in the grip of an extreme diet is really unhappy about it and is crying out for help (under her breath, as it were). Although the need for intervention is not as clear-cut as when there is a threat to life and health, when I have encountered this situation, I have frequently, but not always, felt duty-bound to step in.

Often it doesn't take much effort to start a change. Debra's case is a good example. She had been a vegan for nearly ten years. Once, I suspect, she had embraced this path with enthusiasm, but over the years it had become a mournful duty. She often spoke of the burden of her diet and wished she "were someone else, who didn't have to be so strict about diet." The only reason she stayed vegan, it seemed, was that someone had convinced her long ago that it was immoral to eat anything but plants. She felt hemmed in by guilt, and while she complained constantly about not being able to eat anything that anyone else ate, she saw no possibility of change. In short, she looked like an orthorexic almost ready to step forward, but held back by the force of guilt.

It was really easy to help her break free. I pointed out that no primal peoples known on the face of the earth had ever been vegan, and that the whole idea was really an invention of people who lived in Western countries and had too much time on their hands. I also pointed out that since animals all over the earth devote themselves to eating each other, it could hardly be a violation of natural law for humans to eat animal products, too. (I even made the case that it was an arrogant violation of natural law to try to do so.) As soon as the logical argument behind her diet had been removed, she gave in to her own earnest desires and added a small amount of dairy products and fish to her diet.

It was quite a small change, really, but it was enough to relax her sense of dietary restriction considerably, and it probably improved both her physical and mental health.

When someone admits that he or she would like to quit an extreme diet but can't

Closely related to the preceding situation, this reason for intervention can be summarized as "If a person asks for help, you are justified in giving it." Individuals in this situation begin a conversation by saying, "I wish I could be less obsessed about food." Even if they go on to contradict themselves, I consider this a direct request for help.

However, prior to the publication of my article on orthorexia, not one of my patients ever directly asked me for help with escaping the clutches of an extreme diet. On the contrary, they usually wanted me to tell them to eat in an even more restricted way. I hope that this book will cause more people to understand that a radical diet is not an undiluted virtue and to seek professional assistance.

When it seems that a third party is involved, creating what amounts to a dietary cult

Greg seemed to me to have fallen for a dietary cult. He worked at an agricultural commune headed by a spiritual leader who appeared to be sleeping with all the young women who lived there (a bad sign). According to the leader, any food other than rice, vegetables, and tofu promoted excessive sexual desire. Apparently he believed that only *he* should have any sexual desire, because he required his male followers to adhere to this diet, while he ate plenty of meat.

Greg actually came to me for treatment of digestive discomfort. The more I learned, the more it seemed to me that the commune leader was a real problem. It turned out that he had declared himself doctor of everyone in the commune as well, and whenever anyone became sick, he prescribed additional food deprivation. Furthermore, if any member occasionally failed to follow a dietary rule and was caught, he'd be shamed in front of the community.

I rapidly came to believe that Greg's physical distress was the product of complete suppression of his individuality. It took a great deal of tact and persistence to challenge the leader's hold over Greg's life, but once I had done so, Greg rapidly found his own way.

Fighting orthorexia had really turned out to involve reclaiming individuality.

Of course, it isn't always easy to distinguish between a cult and a legitimate belief. I'd like to think that I would have recognized Jonestown as a cult and that equally I would not regard a major world religion as one. But there are intermediate situations that really aren't clear.

Is macrobiotics a cult? Is raw-foodism one? I don't know. But clearly certain extreme diets with charismatic leaders closely resemble cults, and in those cases intervention certainly does seem appropriate.

When a diet seems to have become an emotional illness

As I discussed in Chapter 3, sometimes orthorexia truly begins to resemble an emotional illness. It may become as insistent as obsessive-compulsive disorder, or as gloomy and self-punishing as major depression. Furthermore, emotional illnesses can appear in the form of orthorexia.

If someone *feels* emotionally ill to you, but on the surface seems to be only following a diet, I recommend that you consider acting on your impression. If you are a layperson, consult a professional. If you are a professional, make sure you are not just reacting in a knee-jerk way to a dietary belief you don't share. However, if you really sense an emotional illness, respond to it as one.

WHEN SHOULD YOU AVOID INTERVENING?

There is an opposite point to keep in mind as well. As I mentioned earlier, many of us have an in-built tendency to criticize other people's food beliefs. Vegetarians were vilified as crazed socialists for decades, and in certain circles in the seventies you could easily devastate someone by calling him a "yogurt eater." There's something about diet that arouses emotional reactions on either side, among both the committed diet followers and the "hang it all, I'll eat anything" nonbelievers.

The fact that you dislike the way someone eats is not sufficient reason for intervening. Look at your own motivations. If you feel a rising urge to insult someone's diet, stop for a moment before you do or say anything. Make sure there really is a good reason to step in.

George is a fairly well known psychotherapist who also pays quite a bit of attention to his own diet. He eats a lot of fruits and vegetables, focuses on whole grains, and consumes very little red meat or dairy products. To him, reducing cholesterol and lowering risk of heart disease is the main purpose of healthy diet, and the way he eats follows current mainstream recommendations on the subject.

Twenty years ago his diet would have been cause for ridicule, but George didn't know that when he explained to me over lunch the disapproval he felt for one of his patients. "The guy is a total vegetarian," he said, "and won't eat any fat at all. He's obsessed. I think it's all about rejecting the mother figure. He thinks he's so virtuous for the way he eats, but to me it's so transparent it makes me want to puke."

My first thought was that George might be getting close to needing a new career. When psychotherapists start to scorn their patients, it's a bad sign. And it was a bit ludicrous. It seemed from what he said that George's patient was following the Pritikin diet, a perfectly good, if rather intense program that can actually reverse heart disease. He was really doing just what George was doing, only more so! Of course, maybe he was just projecting a mother figure onto food, maybe he was symbolically denying himself nurturance, but George's certainty about it was inappropriate.

Of course, the only reason I recognized it so readily was that I've done the same thing. It's very easy to condemn another person's diet. A health care professional or a friend or relative needs to calm down a bit before doing so. Don't judge another person's diet unless you are quite sure on quiet reflection that you really need to. Someone can even eat a rather extreme diet, but if it isn't dangerous and the person seems perfectly happy with that life choice, none of us has a right to interfere—not unless we wish to invite the world to criticize all of *our* life choices.

IF YOU DECIDE TO INTERVENE, HOW SHOULD YOU GO ABOUT IT?

Once identifying that someone's orthorexia is severe enough to warrant stepping outside the norms of personal freedom and making an intervention, the next question is how to do it. The answer: very thoughtfully.

Like all belief systems, orthorexia has defenses built into it. If you attack them head-on, the orthorexic will simply judge you an infidel and refuse to take anything you say seriously. You will seem like someone who doesn't know anything about health, a heathen to be converted rather than an adviser to be trusted.

The first step is to establish trust. It often takes an orthorexic to convince another orthorexic to relax, because only someone who's been there really understands. You have to show that you understand the motivations that underlie extreme diets and that you validate the basic intention behind them. For example, you need to acknowledge that the standard American diet is lousy, that diet can be a powerful force for health, that achieving self-discipline regarding food is an impressive accomplishment, that medical doctors usually don't put enough emphasis on diet—in short, that a reasonable person might very well make large dietary changes and deserve credit for doing so.

Once you've established this basic respect and understanding, you then have to set to work very gradually. You have to gently loosen the grip of self-righteousness and the seduction of extremism. Only when the orthorexic begins to glimpse the possibility that not all goals accomplished at great effort are worth accomplishing and that loosening up on diet might at times be more virtuous than turning the screw tighter do you have a chance of making a difference.

Try telling stories of your own dietary extremism, using a bit of gentle self-mockery to release the death grip. Or maybe you need to come at it from the side, extolling the virtues of spontaneity and psychological freedom. You can be tricky and try to make an alternative food trip look good, if it seems like a step in the right direction.

Of course, you could also share this book.

Sometimes a person is under the spell of a health care professional who seems to be egging her on to further feats of dietary rigor. Many alternative practitioners possess an excessively enthusiastic view of orthorexia. After all, it is perfectly acceptable in most alternative medicine circles to heap shame and ridicule on a person who drinks two cups of coffee a day and has ice cream on Friday nights. The field suffers from an unfortunate lack of holism in this regard!

If you are a health care professional, consider calling up the practitioner and using a variation on the following speech: "I under-stand that you are seeing X and recommending that she carefully control her diet. She feels that it is improving her health consider-ably." (This sentence will ensure that the health care professional doesn't become defensive.)

"I am very glad you've helped her so much. I do have one con-cern, however. Frankly, she's gotten obsessive-compulsive about it. Is there any way you could help her relax a little? From a holistic point of view, I think this is an important perspective to take. The stress can't be good for her."

By invoking inviolable principles of natural medicine (holism, reducing stress) you will make it difficult for the practitioner to ig-nore the message completely. I've seen it work marvelously, although it isn't a sure thing.

Whatever you do, keep in mind that diet is a highly charged subject. It's difficult for people to stop obsessing over food. The sub-ject requires tact, humor, and gentleness, and you might not suc-ceed. But if you can help someone to relax and eat easily again, you've done that person a genuine favor.

Contact Us with Your Story

Do you have a story about orthorexia? A new insight?

What have you found helped you overcome your obsession with healthy food?

E-mail us your stories, successes, strategies, and ideas, at

stories@orthorexia.com

Be sure to include a way to contact you, so we can ask permission to use what you send.

Printed in the United States
by Baker & Taylor Publisher Services